8 Conditions Primary Care Clinicians Dread to Treat

Nataliya Pilipenko • Krishna M. Desai
Editors

8 Conditions Primary Care Clinicians Dread to Treat

A Practical Guide to Nonpharmacological Care

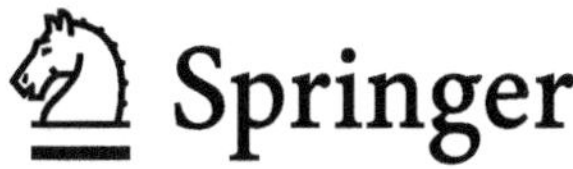

Editors
Nataliya Pilipenko
Center for Family and Community Medicine, Department of Medicine
Columbia University Irving Medical Center/New York Presbyterian Hospital
New York, NY, USA

Department of Psychiatry, Columbia University Irving Medical Center
New York, NY, USA

Krishna M. Desai
Center for Family and Community Medicine
Department of Medicine
Columbia University Irving Medical Center/New York Presbyterian Hospital
New York, NY, USA

Center for Neuroinflammatory and Somatic Disorders
Department of Psychiatry
Columbia University Irving Medical Center
New York, NY, USA

ISBN 978-3-032-12818-8 ISBN 978-3-032-12819-5 (eBook)
https://doi.org/10.1007/978-3-032-12819-5

This Springer imprint is published by the registered company Springer Nature Switzerland AG
The registered company address is: Gewerbestrasse 11, 6330 Cham, Switzerland

Contents

Chapter 1
Introduction

Nataliya Pilipenko and Krishna M. Desai

Introduction

Despite significant technological advances and the astronomical costs of healthcare, patient outcomes in the U.S. remain suboptimal [19]. Furthermore, ongoing efforts to address healthcare disparities result in growing pressure to incorporate a broader range of interventions and techniques to improve illness control and promote health. As affordable and effective healthcare remains elusive [10] nonpharmacological interventions (**NPIs**) are receiving increased attention and interest [4].

Role of Primary Care in the Healthcare Delivery

Primary care (**PC**) is "the provision of integrated, accessible health care services by physicians and their health care teams … addressing a large majority of personal health care needs, developing a sustained partnership with patients, and practicing in the context of family and community" [1]. **PC**'s structure is effectively summarized by the 4Cs model: it is the point for patients' first **c**ontact with the

N. Pilipenko (✉)
Center for Family and Community Medicine, Department of Medicine, Columbia University Irving Medical Center/New York Presbyterian Hospital, New York, NY, USA

Department of Psychiatry, Columbia University Irving Medical Center, New York, NY, USA
e-mail: np2615@cumc.columbia.edu

K. M. Desai
Center for Family and Community Medicine, Department of Medicine, Columbia University Irving Medical Center/New York Presbyterian Hospital, New York, NY, USA

Center for Neuroinflammatory and Somatic Disorders, Department of Psychiatry, Columbia University Irving Medical Center, New York, NY, USA

N. Pilipenko, K. M. Desai (eds.), *8 Conditions Primary Care Clinicians Dread to Treat*, https://doi.org/10.1007/978-3-032-12819-5_1

medical system, provides care **c**ontinuity, offers **c**omprehensive care, and delivers care **c**oordination to address multiple needs [20]. Despite ongoing concerns about **PC**'s accessibility, it is substantially utilized in the U.S., with over half a million visits completed annually [5]. Furthermore, **PC** is known as the nation's "de facto mental healthcare service" [11] as many patients with psychiatric needs receive care only in this setting. Thus, PC physicians may be uniquely positioned to deliver care to diverse populations experiencing a broad spectrum of healthcare needs and play a central role in bridging population health gaps.

Delivering Patient Centered Care

Patient-centered care (**PCC**), also known as person-centered care, is defined as "respectful and responsive to individual patient preferences, needs, and values [thus] ensuring that patient values guide all clinical decisions" [23, p. 6]. Although **PCC** is at the heart of healthcare care improvement efforts for over a decade, its implementation remains challenging. While individual physicians have limited control over the system-level barriers to **PCC** delivery, they have significant leverage in implementation of concrete **PCC** activities within their day-to-day patient care. Specifically, dimensions of **PCC delivery** include: biopsychosocial perspective, "patient-as-person," sharing power and responsibility, therapeutic alliance, and "doctor-as-person" [13].

Thus, **PCC** relies on competent use of **NPI**s (necessary for biopsychosocial care) as well as effective management of patient-physician relationships. Both components require practical skills which are grounded in understanding of both contextualized and **culturally competent care**.

Contextualized Care

Contextualized medical care includes "life circumstances and patient behaviors relevant to planning a particular patient's care" [24]. Contextual factors include a broad range of circumstances and behaviors which can be both intrinsic (e.g. illness attitudes, health behaviors, emotional states) or external (e.g. finances, environment, access to care). Contextual factors may be elicited by asking: "What kinds of things are essential to know [about this patient] in order to provide appropriate care?" [25, p. 21].

Unfortunately, within the current model of medical care delivery and training, patients are often "perceived as someone upon whom a set of tasks must be efficiently completed, rather than as a person with whom [physician] seeks to engage with a sense of shared humanity" [25, p. 21]. However, research indicates that contextual care skills can be significantly improved leading to both better illness outcomes and reduced healthcare costs [26].

Culturally Competent Care

Culture is the "integrated patterns of learned beliefs and behaviors that can be shared among groups and include thoughts, styles of communicating, ways of interacting, views on roles and relationships, values, practices, and customs" [3]. As the US population is becoming increasingly racially and ethnically diverse, [21] there is growing recognition that the heterogeneity and complexity of patients' lives must be taken into consieration for effective delivery of **PCC**.

Efforts towards holistic yet nuanced understanding of patients' experiences can be understood via intersectionality framework, which proposes that multifaceted categories (including but not limited to race, class and gender) are continuously interacting to inform unique personal experience [9]. Intersectionality challenges historical efforts to improve physician's cultural competence by teaching "do's and don'ts" of working with discrete ethnic and cultural groups since such approach promulgates further stereotyping (see [2] for further discussion). Therefore, awareness and utilization of culturally informed interviewing frameworks can significantly assist physicians in delivering **PCC**. Specifically, Betancourt [2] offers an efficient and elegant ESFT model which aligns with **PCC** goals and provides clear questions to guide inquiry.

In this chapter, we introduce concepts of ***Culturally Competent Care*** and ***Contextualized Care*** as both are centrally important to the overarching implementation of **PCC**. Understanding of these concepts is necessary for effective management of all conditions discussed in this book. Furthermore, while we aim to provide clear language for speaking with patients about the specific conditions in each chapter. Each **PC** visit should be grounded in effective communication practices, including: clear shared understanding of goals via agenda setting, effective elicitation of patient's experiences and perspectives (via application of ***Culturally Competent Care*** and ***Contextualized Care*** principles and techniques), shared decision making, and clear agreement on the post visit plans confirmed via teach back. Table 1.1 presents resources to support development of relevant skills and competencies.

What Is Integrative Medicine?

Integrative medicine (**IM**) is an approach that emphasizes a whole-person framework and prioritizes establishing a therapeutic alliance with the patient. **IM** includes all aspects of the lifestyle and makes use of all appropriate evidence-based therapies, which include complementary therapies alongside conventional therapies.

Key **IM** interventions include Lifestyle Medicine (LM), herbs/botanicals/supplements (HBS), mind-body practices (MBPs) and elements of non-allopathic systems of medicine such as acupuncture from Traditional Chinese Medicine. These key interventions are introduced below. Please refer to materials in Table 1.1 for a more in-depth understanding of these and other **IM** techniques.

Lifestyle Medicine (LM)

LM is an evidence-based medical specialty that focuses on treating chronic conditions by applying therapeutic lifestyle interventions [1]. This approach incorporates comprehensive and detailed assessment of six main lifestyle factors: nutrition, physical activity, stress, quality of sleep, social connections, and use of substances [12]. Since poor nutrition, nonrestorative sleep, chronic stress, physical inactivity, and substance use are contributors to, and amplifiers of, a wide range of somatic symptoms [6], addressing these areas can have profound effects on symptom burden.

Herbs, Botanicals, and Supplements (HBS)

Herbs are plants or components of plants (leaves, flowers, stems, roots, seeds, or bark) used for their therapeutic properties. Botanicals are a broader category encompassing any product derived from plants used for therapeutic purposes. This term includes herbs but also extends to plant-derived metabolites, essential oils, and compounds used in dietary supplements or topical preparations. Dietary supplements are products intended to augment the diet and may contain one or more ingredients such as vitamins, minerals, amino acids, herbs, or other botanicals [16].

Prescribing HBS requires careful clinical considerations to ensure safe use. Specifically, physicians must consider cost, safety, side effects, HBS-drug interactions, patient's comorbidities, formulations, reputability and third-party testing of products being recommended. All of these considerations should be discussed with the patient to ensure safe and appropriate use. Consumerlab.com and Natural Medicines Comprehensive Database are important resources for physicians who recommend HBS as both sites provide information about critical considerations when recommending HBS. Furthermore, Good Manufacturing Practice (GMP) and Natural Standard Foundation (NSF) labels on products can alert patients and physicians that the product is of higher quality and was third party tested.

Mind-Body Practices (MBPs)

MBPs are a large and diverse group of procedures or techniques that target brain-body interactions to promote health [14]. Although MBPs are generally safe, accessible, and well tolerated, physicians should be aware of potential risks of these approaches. Specifically, MBPs involve focused attention on bodily sensations and thoughts, which may, in some cases, intensify distressing experiences. Thus, physicians interested in including MBPs, should consider seeking training and consultation to ensure competent implementation and to navigate challenges and risks that may arise.

Although the popularity of MBPs is growing along with evidence to support their use, further research is needed to identify which patient groups may experience the most benefit. Furthermore, it is important to recognize that **IM** should not replace any standard of care medical treatments. Rather, **IM** therapies are incorporated into multifaceted treatment plans that are grounded in best available evidence, safety considerations, patient preferences, and cost-effectiveness.

The following MBPs will be discussed in this book [8, 18].

1. *Mindfulness-based stress reduction (MBSR):* mindfulness practices originated from Buddhism. The gold standard of MBSR is Jon Kabat-Zinn's (1979) eight-week MBSR program which combined mindfulness meditation, body awareness, and gentle movement that was aimed at reducing stress, pain, and managing a range of chronic diseases.
2. *Meditation*: variety of contemplative practices and techniques that involve regulating the mind and body through a heightened state of awareness.
3. *Guided Imagery*: a technique that uses focused visualization, often imagining calming or healing scenes, or desired outcomes to improve symptoms and support behavior changes.
4. *Biofeedback*: a method that utilizes physiological measurements (e.g. heart rate, muscle contractions, skin temperature) to regulate physical and mental processes.
5. *Hypnosis*: induced state of consciousness in which an individual has heightened focus and suggestibility.
6. *Yoga*: an ancient practice originating from India, that combines physical postures (asanas), breathing (pranayama), and meditation (dhyana).
7. *Breathwork*: Intentional regulation of breathing patterns to influence physiological or psychological states.

Acupuncture

Acupuncture originated from Traditional Chinese Medicine and uses very small needles that are inserted into the skin and either manually or electronically stimulated. From an Eastern view, it balances Qi ("Chi"); biomedically, it triggers micro-trauma that promotes neurotransmitter release, reduces inflammation, suppresses pain signaling, and activates endogenous opioids. Neuroimaging shows modulation of pain-related brain networks via acupuncture [15].

Effectiveness depends on needle technique, acupoint selection, and practitioner expertise. Generally, acupuncture is considered safe however patients should be referred to licensed providers and informed of mild side effects (soreness, minor bleeding) and rare risks (infection, nerve injury). Caution should be practiced when referring patients with fear of needles or those who may be immunocompromised. Those fearful of needles may prefer acupressure, a needle-free, low-risk alternative that can be self-administered. It should be noted that although the body of evidence is promising, studies are limited by varying methodological quality, small sample sizes, and publication bias. Further research efforts are warranted to evaluate the effectiveness of acupuncture for a variety of conditions.

Behavior Change

It is important for physicians to recognize that behavior change necessary for **IM** implementation is inherently challenging. Thus, physicians should employ effective communication skills to engage patients as partners in promoting healthy behaviors (see Delivering Patient Centered Care for further discussion).

Health Care Disparities

The American Medical Association (2016) highlights the importance of physicians' role in addressing health disparities. Thus, it is critical to acknowledge broader social and structural factors which actively shape health and illness experiences of each patient. Furthermore, physicians should advocate for structural solutions that promote health equity and support sustainable improvements in the health of patients they serve.

Our Perspective: Challenges to PCC in PC

For almost 10 years, editors of this book have co-led an **IM** consultation service based within a community-based **PC** clinic. Over time, we observed a pattern which appears to contribute to ongoing poor management of multiple conditions. Specifically, although **PC** physicians acknowledge the role of psychosocial and behavioral factors in physical and psychiatric illnesses, they are often ill-prepared to accurately diagnose and address specifics of condition-related concerns. Instead, they rely on pharmacotherapies and specialty referrals. This can leave patients frustrated and fearful as symptoms persist, prompting repeated visits for diagnostic clarification and treatment. Physicians, in turn, order more tests, make additional referrals, and prescribe more medications—all of which increase costs, risks of side effects, and incidental findings without improving health. Moreover, patients may forgo referrals and decline treatment recommendations for reasons ranging from distrust of medications to financial constraints. Synergistically, these behaviors contribute to ineffective care, high costs, and ongoing distrust of the medical professionals.

This book aims to address existing gaps in knowledge and skills by providing clear, practical, and succinct guidance to physicians. It focuses on eight common psychiatric and chronic pain conditions which require **non-pharmacological interventions** for sustained symptom improvement.

We encourage physicians to partner with interdisciplinary colleagues to create integrative, team-based models of care that better serve the needs of their patients than traditional time limited office visits. This approach is particularly important for patients with complex psychosocial needs and systemic barriers to accessing holistic, high-quality care.

Who Is This Book For?

This book focuses on the needs of **PC** physicians and trainees. However, we hope that our work can be useful to all clinicians who encounter these eight conditions in their work.

What Is Covered?

This book includes eight chapters addressing conditions which require **non-pharmacological interventions** for successful symptom management. First four chapters (Chaps. 2, 3, 4, and 5), focus on psychiatric conditions: somatic symptom disorder/illness anxiety disorder, panic disorder, posttraumatic stress disorder, and insomnia. Subsequent four chapters (Chaps. 6, 7, 8, and 9) address pain-related conditions including: chronic pain, irritable bowel syndrome, fibromyalgia, and headache.

Each chapter includes the following sections:

1. Brief diagnostic description
2. Review of prevalence, risk factors, disparities pertaining to the specific condition
3. Symptom assessment and screening tools. This section includes information about measure's structure, scoring, psychometric properties, accessibility and other pertient factors. Additionally, it includes information about each tool's availability in five languages which are most spoken in the U.S.—Spanish, Chinese, Tagalog, Vietnamese, Arabic [22].
4. Nonpharmacological conceptualization of the condition. Specific education for the patient is included under the "Message" section, while rationale and relevant literature are presented under the "Why?" section.
5. Overview of non-pharmacological techniques which physicians can utilize during visit to improve specific condition's symptoms and management.
6. Condition-relevant **IM** interventions and techniques
7. Clinical pearls
8. Frequently asked patient questions as well as response recommendations.
9. A case vignette is included in each chapter to illustrate key points.
10. A list of patient education resources.

The final chapter (Chap. 10) offers an overview of non-pharmacological psychotherapies. The primary goal of this chapter is to help **PC** physicians understand the process by which evidence-based psychotherapies work thus equipping them for both interprofessional collaborations and patient advocacy.

Table 1.1 Supporting resources

Title	Description
Clinical Interviewing	
Frankel., R.M., & Stein, T. (1999). Getting the most out of the clinical encounter: The Four Habits Model. The Permanente Journal, 3(3).	Article presents important clinical interviewing tasks, provides rationale for these and outlines practical steps to supporting PCC
Fortin, A., Dwamena, F., Frankel, R.M., & Smith, R.C. (2012). Smith's patient centered interviewing: An evidence-based method. (3rd Ed.) New York: McGraw-Hill.	Book outlines Smith's interviewing model and presents detailed description of biopsychosocially-grounded inquiry
Epstein, R.M., Mauksch, L., Carroll, J., & Jaen, C.R. (2008). Have you really addressed your patient's concerns? *Family Practice Management*. Retrieved from: www.aafp.org/fpm	Article addresses agenda setting skills
Pilipenko, N., & Chang, M. N. (2024). Re-imagining clinical interviewing: Bridging the gap between theory and practice for equitable care. In E. Bonilla-Silva, E. Haozous, G. Kayingo, W. McDade, L. Meeks, A. Núñez, T. Oyeyemi, J. Southerland, & J. Sukhera (Eds.), Reimagining medical education for the future of health equity and social justice (pp. 140–154). Elsevier.	Chapter outlines specific interviewing behaviors to support PCC—including agenda setting, integrating medical health record, interviewing techniques, working with interpreters, and working with patient companions.
Culturally Informed Interviewing—ESFM Model	
Betancourt, J.R. (2006). Cultural competency: Providing quality care to diverse populations. Consultant Pharmacist, 21, 988–995.	Article outlines rationale behind culturally informed interviewing and outlines ESFT model.
Betancourt JR, Carrillo JE, & Green AR. (1999) Hypertension in Multicultural and Minority Populations: Linking Communication to Compliance. *Current Hypertension Reports, 1*(6), 482–488.	The article illustrates the role of culturally-informed illness conceptualization and result on illness management.
Contextualized Care	
Weiner, M., & Schwartz, A. (2023). Listening for what matters: Avoiding contextual errors in health care (2nd ed.). Oxford University Press.	The book outlines rationale, research and application of contextualized care.
Weiner, S., et al., (2020). Evaluation of a patient-collected audio audit and feedback quality improvement program on clinician attention to patient life context and health care costs in the Veterans Affairs Health Care System. JAMA Network Open, 3(7), e209644. https://doi.org/10.1001/jamanetworkopen.2020.9644	Article outlines research supporting the utility of contextualized care for cost reduction and health improvement.
Integrative Medicine	
Rakel, D. P., & Minichiello, V. J. (2023). *Integrative medicine* (5th ed.). Elsevier.	This book is a comprehensive reference text book for the clinical application of evidence based integrative therapies.
American College of Lifestyle Medicine https://lifestylemedicine.org	The American College of Lifestyle Medicine (ACLM) website is a comprehensive resource for physicians that provides evidence based LM tools for clinical practice.

(continued)

Table 1.1 (continued)

Clinical Interviewing	
Title	Description
Natural Medicines Comprehensive Database https://naturalmedicines.therapeuticresearch.com	A subscription-based, evidence-based reference resource for unbiased, clinically useful data on efficacy, safety, interactions, dosing, and quality of natural products such as herbs, botanicals, and supplements.
Consumerlab.com	A private, independent organization that tests and evaluates natural products. It is designed to help consumers and healthcare professionals identify high-quality products through independent testing and analysis.
Dr. Andrew Weil's website https://www.drweil.com/	A resource for education and information for patients and healthcare professionals, based on the principles of integrative medicine.
Body of Wonder podcast https://awcim.arizona.edu/body_of_wonder.html	Podcast of the University of Arizona Andrew Weil Center for Integrative Medicine for patients and healthcare professionals focused on IM topics.
Mindful Leader https://www.mindfulleader.org/	An accredited training provider through International Accreditors of Continuing Education and Training (IACET) that provides Mindfulness-Based Stress Reduction courses and events.
Palouse Mindfulness https://palousemindfulness.com/	A 501(c)3 non-profit organization that provides a free online MBSR course and resources for patients and healthcare professionals.
National Center for Complementary and Integrative Health https://www.nccih.nih.gov/	Conducts research and provides information about complementary health products and practices.
Additional Resources: Specialty Literature	
First, M. B. (Ed.). (2023). DSM-5-TR® handbook of differential diagnosis. American Psychiatric Association Publishing. https://doi.org/10.1176/appi.books.9781615375363	Handbook offers effective guidance for differentially diagnosing psychiatric disorders

References

1. American Academy of Family Physicians. Primary care. Available at: https://www.aafp.org/about/policies/all/primary-care.html.
2. Betancourt JR. Cultural competency: providing quality care to diverse populations. Consult Pharm. 2006;21(11):988–95. https://doi.org/10.4140/TCP.n.2006.988.
3. Betancourt JR, Green AR, Carrillo JE. Cultural competence in health care: emerging frameworks and practical approaches. 2002. The Commonwealth Fund https://www.commonwealthfund.org/publications/fund-reports/2002/oct/cultural-competence-health-care-emerging-frameworks-and.
4. Castellano-Tejedor C. Non-pharmacological interventions for the management of chronic health conditions and non-communicable diseases. Int J Environ Res Public Health. 2022;19(14):8536. https://doi.org/10.3390/ijerph19148536.
5. Centers for Disease Control and Prevention. National Ambulatory Medical Care Survey: 2019 national summary tables. U.S. Department of Health and Human Services. 2021. https://www.cdc.gov/nchs/data/ahcd/namcs_summary/2019-namcs-web-tables-508.pdf.
6. Creed F. The risk factors for self-reported fibromyalgia with and without multiple somatic symptoms: The Lifelines cohort study. J Psychosom Res. 2022;155:110745. https://doi.org/10.1016/j.jpsychores.2022.110745.
7. First MB, editor. DSM-5-TR® handbook of differential diagnosis. American Psychiatric Association Publishing; 2023. https://doi.org/10.1176/appi.books.9781615375363.
8. Freeman M, Ayers C, Kondo K, Noonan K, O'Neil M, Morasco B, Kansagara D. Guided imagery, biofeedback, and hypnosis: a map of the evidence. 2019. (VA ESP project #05–225).
9. Guittar SG, Guittar NA. Intersectionality. In: Wright JD, editor. International encyclopedia of the social & behavioral sciences. 2nd ed. Elsevier; 2015. p. 657–62. https://doi.org/10.1016/B978-0-08-097086-8.10558-1.
10. Hostetter J, Schwarz N, Klug M, Wynne J, Basson MD. Primary care visits increase utilization of evidence-based preventative health measures. BMC Fam Pract. 2020;21(1):151. https://doi.org/10.1186/s12875-020-01216-8.
11. Kessler R, Stafford D. Primary care is the de facto mental health system. In: Kessler R, Stafford D, editors. Collaborative medicine case studies: evidence in practice. Springer; 2008. p. 9–2.
12. Lippman D, Stump M, Veazey E, Guimarães ST, Rosenfeld R, Kelly JH, Ornish D, Katz DL. Foundations of lifestyle medicine and its evolution. Mayo Clin Proc Innov Qual Outcomes. 2024;8(1):97–111. https://doi.org/10.1016/j.mayocpiqo.2023.11.004.
13. Mead N, Bower P. Patient-centredness: a conceptual framework and review of the empirical literature. Soc Sci Med. 2000;51(7):1087–110. https://doi.org/10.1016/S0277-9536(00)00098-8.
14. National Center for Complementary and Integrative Health. Mind and body practices. U.S. Department of Health and Human Services, National Institutes of Health. 2025. https://www.nccih.nih.gov/health/mind-and-body-practices.
15. Niruthisard S, Ma Q, Napadow V. Recent advances in acupuncture for pain relief. Pain Rep. 2024;9(5):e1188. Published 2024 Sep 13. https://doi.org/10.1097/PR9.0000000000001188.
16. Office of Dietary Supplements. Botanical dietary supplements background information: fact sheet for consumers. U.S. Department of Health & Human Services, National Institutes of Health. 2020. https://ods.od.nih.gov/factsheets/BotanicalBackground-Consumer/.
17. Pilipenko N, Chang MN. Re-imagining clinical interviewing: bridging the gap between theory and practice for equitable care. In: Bonilla-Silva E, Haozous E, Kayingo G, McDade W, Meeks L, Núñez A, Oyeyemi T, Southerland J, Sukhera J, editors. Reimagining medical education for the future of health equity and social justice. Elsevier; 2024. p. 140–54.
18. Saoji AA, Raghavendra BR, Manjunath NK. Effects of yogic breath regulation: a narrative review of scientific evidence. J Ayurveda Integr Med. 2019;10(1):50–8. https://doi.org/10.1016/j.jaim.2017.07.008.
19. Schneider EC, Shah A, Doty MM, Tikkanen R, Fields K, Williams RD. Mirror, mirror 2021: reflecting poorly—health care in the U.S. compared to other high-income countries. The

Commonwealth Fund. 2023. https://www.commonwealthfund.org/sites/default/files/2021-08/Schneider_Mirror_Mirror_2021.pdf.
20. Starfield B, Shi L, Macinko J. Contribution of primary care to health systems and health. Milbank Q. 2005;83(3):457–502. https://doi.org/10.1111/j.1468-0009.2005.00409.x.
21. U.S. Census Bureau. 2020 United States population more racially and ethnically diverse than 2010. 2021. https://www.census.gov/library/stories/2021/08/2020-united-states-population-more-racially-ethnically-diverse-than-2010.html.
22. U.S. Census Bureau. Languages we speak in the United States. 2022. https://www.census.gov/library/stories/2022/12/languages-we-speak-in-united-states.html.
23. U.S. Department of Health and Human Services. The health consequences of smoking—50 years of progress: A report of the Surgeon General (Publication No. NBK222274). Centers for Disease Control and Prevention, National Center for Chronic Disease Prevention and Health Promotion, Office on Smoking and Health. 2014. https://www.ncbi.nlm.nih.gov/books/NBK222274/.
24. Weiner SJ, Schwartz A, Weaver F, Goldberg J, Yudkowsky R, Sharma G, Binns-Calvey A, Preyss B, Schapira MM, Persell SD, Jacobs E, Abrams RI. Contextual errors and failures in individualizing patient care: a multicenter study. Ann Intern Med. 2010;153(2):69–75. https://doi.org/10.7326/0003-4819-153-2-201007200-00002.
25. Weiner M, Schwartz A. Listening for what matters: avoiding contextual errors in health care. 2nd ed. Oxford University Press; 2023.
26. Weiner S, Schwartz A, Altman L, Ball S, Bartle B, Binns-Calvey A, Chan C, Falck-Ytter C, Frenchman M, Gee B, Jackson JL, Jordan N, Kass B, Kelly B, Safdar N, Scholcoff C, Sharma G, Weaver F, Wopat M. Evaluation of a patient-collected audio audit and feedback quality improvement program on clinician attention to patient life context and health care costs in the Veterans Affairs Health Care System. JAMA Netw Open. 2020;3(7):e209644. https://doi.org/10.1001/jamanetworkopen.2020.9644.

Part I
Psychiatric Conditions

Chapter 2
Somatic Symptom Disorder and Illness Anxiety Disorder

Nataliya Pilipenko, Krishna M. Desai, and Aury Garcia

Case Vignette: Part 1

Ms. M is a 45-year-old woman with a history of hypertension and asthma presenting to see Dr. A.

Ms. M.: *I have not been feeling well. For the last seven months I have been dealing with horrible stomach pain, back pain, and foamy urine. I am worried that I may die from cancer, and no one is listening to me!*

Dr. A: *You sound very concerned. I see in your chart that you went to the emergency department (ED) three times in the last month with these issues. Can you tell me what has been done to address your symptoms?*

Ms. M: *Every time I go to the ED, they tell me that my physical exam, blood work, and imaging are all normal. They just can't figure it out. So frustrating! I have seen so many doctors! I got a colonoscopy, that was normal. I am taking medication for constipation. I have done elimination diets. Tried warm compresses, lidocaine patches, Tylenol, and Ibuprofen. I tried everything!*

N. Pilipenko (✉)
Center for Family and Community Medicine, Department of Medicine, Columbia University Irving Medical Center/New York Presbyterian Hospital, New York, NY, USA

Department of Psychiatry, Columbia University Irving Medical Center, New York, NY, USA
e-mail: np2615@cumc.columbia.edu

K. M. Desai
Center for Family and Community Medicine, Department of Medicine, Columbia University Irving Medical Center/New York Presbyterian Hospital, New York, NY, USA

Center for Neuroinflammatory and Somatic Disorders, Department of Psychiatry, Columbia University Irving Medical Center, New York, NY, USA

A. Garcia
Center for Family and Community Medicine, Department of Medicine, Columbia University Irving Medical Center/New York Presbyterian Hospital, New York, NY, USA

N. Pilipenko, K. M. Desai (eds.), *8 Conditions Primary Care Clinicians Dread to Treat*, https://doi.org/10.1007/978-3-032-12819-5_2

Dr. A. *So, these symptoms have been going on for some time now, lots of tests have been run, lots of medications tried, but there seems to be no specific cause nor a cure. I know you mentioned being worried about cancer, what is your understanding of the tests so far?*

Ms. M: *I know that tests do not show cancer. When I get tested and the test is normal, I do feel a little better. Even my pain seems a little less. But then some days I am so worried I must take days off work and I stay in bed and cry because I am so scared! I just can't stop thinking about my stomach pain. I have been trying to get myself to stop Googling because it scares me even more.*

Dr. A: *It sounds like your physical symptoms are causing you not only a lot of physical pain but also making you very upset. I think we should plan to approach both your physical symptoms as well as your distress and anxiety about them, because how you feel emotionally also plays an important role in your health and wellbeing.*

At the end of the visit, Dr. A asks Ms. M to complete Patient Health Questionnaire-15 and 14-item (Short) Health Anxiety Inventory (See **Symptom Assessment Tools**). Scores indicate significant prevalence of somatic symptoms as well as high symptom-related distress. Symptom scores are reviewed with Ms. M.

Diagnosis: Brief Description

Somatic Symptom Disorder (**SSD**) diagnosis was first introduced in the fifth edition of the Diagnostic and Statistical Manual of Mental Disorders [5]. This new diagnosis replaced several conditions in the somatoform category (i.e., somatization disorder, somatoform disorder, pain disorder, hypochondriasis). The goal of this change was to shift diagnostic focus away from the "medically unexplained" presentation of physical symptoms, thus promoting holistic conceptualization and care [5, 13]. Per DSM-5-TR [4], while most patients formally diagnosed with hypochondriasis would meet criteria for **SSD**, approximately 30% would meet criteria for Illness Anxiety Disorder (**IAD**) instead (p. 357).

SSD diagnosis requires presence of at least one somatic symptom/concern which is either distressing or results in disruption of functioning. Whether the symptom/concern is medically explained has no bearing on this diagnosis. Additionally, at least one of the following should be present: 1. Excessive/recurring thoughts about seriousness of symptom/concern 2. High symptom/concern-related anxiety 3. Excessive symptom/concern focus. While the physical symptom may not be continuously present, diagnosis of **SSD** requires that the preoccupation is ongoing for at least 6 months. The specifier "with persistent pain" is appropriate to include when **SSD** symptoms are pain focused [4, p. 351].

SSD is differentiated from **IAD**, as the latter is associated with excessive health-related preoccupation (i.e., having or acquiring medical illness) in the absence or only minimal presence of physical symptoms [4, p. 357]. Similarly to **SSD**, IAD is characterized by high anxiety about health, excessive health-related behaviors (e.g., symptom checking), and **avoidance**. Similarly to **SSD**, preoccupation must last at least 6 months, but "specific illness fears may change over time" [4, p. 357].

Please refer to DSM-5-TR [4] for information pertaining to the differential diagnostic considerations for **SSD/IAD**.

Prevalence, Risk Factors, and Disparities

Prevalence rates of **SSD** in the general adult population are estimated as 4–6% [4, p. 353]. In PC, **SSD** may be overrepresented, with estimated rates of 5–35% [23]. Prevalence of **IAD** is estimated as 1.3–10% in the general population and 2.2–8% in the PC (4, p. 358). However, accurate prevalence rates of **SSD/IAD** are challenging to estimate since research largely focuses on "medically unexplained symptoms" or "functional syndromes" rather than excessive symptom-related concerns [35].

SSD symptoms are associated with female gender, anxiety, depression, and presence of medical illnesses. Trauma history, less formal education, lower socioeconomic status, and a recent history of stressful or health-related events are associated with higher **SSD** frequency [4, pp. 353–354]. Similarly, **IAD** may be precipitated by major stressors or illnesses (own or significant others') (4, p. 359).

Furthermore, research examining the role of intersectional inequalities in somatic symptom severity indicates that three groups report the highest symptom burden. Specifically: males with low income whose parent(s) immigrated, females with low income who immigrated themselves, and females with low income and no history of migration [8]. Finally, meta-analysis findings by Barbek et al. [7] reports that persons with higher socioeconomic status have 37% lower prevalence rate of **IAD** compared to those with lower socioeconomic status (*OR* = 0.63, 95%-CI [0.43–0.92]).

Symptom Assessment Tools

Table 2.1 presents two **SSD** and one **IAD** screening tools. The Patient Health Questionnaire -15 [27] and Somatic Symptom Scale-8 (SSS-8, [18]) assess the degree of being "bothered by" physical symptoms. The 14-item (Short) Health Anxiety Inventory (SHAI-14, [39]) assesses cognitive, affective, and behavioral aspects of health anxiety.

Table 2.1 Somatic Symptom and Illness Anxiety Disorder screening tools

Screener name	Items #	Rating scale scoring	Cut offs	Assessment timeline	Availability	Psychometric properties	Non-english versions available?
Patient Health Questionnaire 15 item scale (PHQ-15)	15 [27]	3-point likert [27] 0 = Not bothered at all to 2 = Bothered a lot	5—low [27] 10—medium 15—high Somatic symptom severity	1 week [27]	Open access [27]	Strong association between PHQ-15 scores and functional status, disability days, and symptom-related difficulty measures (convergent validity) [27] Appropriate discriminant validity with depression symptoms screening [27] Specificity and sensitivity equal to 61.9 and 56.5% with cut off score of 9 [12]	Arabic [2], Chinese [44], Spanish [38]
Somatic Symptom Scale 8 (SSS-8)	8 [18]	5-point likert [18] 0 = Not at all to 4 = Very much	0–3—no to [18] minimal 4–7—low 8–11—medium 12–15—high 16–32—very high	1 week [18]	Open access [18]	Good internal consistency (Cronbach $\alpha = .81$) [18] 1 point increase score is associated with 12% increase in health care visits (incidence rate ratio, 1.12 [95% confidence interval: 1.10–1.14]) [18] Factor analysis supports 4 symptom clusters: Gastrointestinal, pain, cardiopulmonary, and fatigue [18]	Chinese [28]
Short Health Anxiety Inventory (SHAI-14)	14 [39]	0–54 [32] Health Anxiety (items 1–14) score = 0–42 Negative consequences of becoming ill (items 15–18) score = 0–12	Higher scores [32] indicate more health anxiety and beliefs of negative consequences of becoming ill	6 months [39]	Open access [39]	Good internal consistency (Cronbach $\alpha = .89$) [39]	Arabic [3], Chinese [43], Spanish [6]

Non-pharmacological Conceptualization: What to Say to the Patient?

Overall, effective care of **SSD/IAD** requires physicians to effectively communicate three key messages:

Message # 1. Health Is Impacted by Complex Interplay of Physical and Mental Processes

Bodily symptoms can be frightening, leading to physical stress response (e.g., racing heart, digestive problems, pain due to muscle tension). Additionally, both worry and attention to the physical symptoms can increase the experience of these symptoms.

Why? This formulation actively focuses on the whole-person/biopsychosocial conceptualization thus avoiding **mind-body** dualism of the biomedical approach, while concurrently validating and communicating empathy for patients' experiences.

Message # 2. Medicine Does Not Have All the Answers

Despite medical advances, up to a half of all physical symptoms may not be explained by modern medicine. Even if the cause of illness is known, complete symptom elimination may be difficult to achieve. Diagnostic tests and procedures may be helpful, however also have risks and may not identify in a specific cause which can be addressed to eliminate suffering.

Why? Limits as well as risks of medical approaches must be explicitly recognized for patient-centered care. Currently 30–50% of symptoms in medical symptoms are unexplained [26, 42].

Furthermore, complications of medical care cannot be ignored. For example, a recent cohort study reported that 38% (95% CI [32.6, 43.4]) of surgical patients experienced complications while 15.8% (95% CI [12.7, 19.0]) experienced major adverse events [14]. Additionally, a scoping review of adverse drug reactions among PC patients reports that these may range from 6–80% [25]. Thus acknowledgments of modern medicine's limits normalizes and models the ubiquitous nature of uncertainty which patients suffering from **SSD/IAD** have difficulties tolerating.

Message #3. Both Physical and Emotional Aspects of Illness Need to Be Addressed

Physical concerns must be addressed and receive full evaluation in line with best practices, however anxiety and distress about physical symptoms have now reached levels (per symptom screening, self-report of symptoms and distress/impairment) which warrant treatment as a separate diagnosis.

Why? Statement formulates **SSD/IAD**-related distress as a treatment goal and links management to overall goals of health improvement. This holistic approach avoids **mind-body** dualism and supports patient-centered care [35].

It is important to highlight physician-level factors which will impede care of patients presenting with **SSD** and **IAD**. These include: lack of full exploration of patients' presenting concerns and failure to understand patients' symptom-related beliefs, failure to provide evidence-based care coupled with vague or ineffective explanations of medical diagnosis/findings, sole focus on biomedical model, poor understanding of **SSD** as a medical diagnosis, and negative attitudes towards patients (e.g. lack of empathy, belief that patient lacks insight or is being "difficult") [31].

Non-pharmacological Treatment Options: What Can Be Done?

Several processes are implicated in etiology and maintenance of **SSD/IAD**. Addressing these can be helpful for improved symptom management. Three processes include: **catastrophizing**, behavioral **avoidance/safety behaviors**, difficulties with tolerating strong **negative emotions**/uncertainty.

1. **Catastrophizing**

Catastrophizing (also known as "fortune telling") is a cognitive process whereby an event, experience or symptom is appraised as an indicator of highly negative future outcome(s) ([9], p 253). See Vignette—Continued for illustration.

At the center of **SSD/IAD** is the patient's appraisal of physical symptoms as dangerous and threatening. **Catastrophizing** maintains patient in a state of high focus on the symptoms along with negative arousal and worry, focusing on the "worst case scenario" mode while ignoring other, more likely and benign possibilities and symptom explanations. **Catastrophizing** is linked to anxiety, possibly via dorsomedial prefrontal cortex [33].

How to Address?

Cognitive disputation technique is a key tool for addressing catastrophic thinking within cognitive behavioral approach.

As the first step, catastrophic thought or statement is identified. Catastrophic beliefs can be elicited by asking: "What is your biggest concern about [symptom]?"

As the second step, the patient is asked to list out all evidence which supports or verifies their thought. Such evidence can include personal anecdotes (e.g. "My aunt had similar symptoms before she was diagnosed with cancer"), beliefs (e.g. "If a symptom is not explained it must be dangerous") or information received from various sources (e.g. "I listened to a podcast which mentioned that rates of stomach cancer is going up and often symptoms are ignored until it's too late"). A complete list of all "evidence" supporting the belief should be created. At this step, no attempt should be made to address these beliefs.

As the third step, the patient is asked to list out all "evidence" which does not support the belief. For example, prior medical testing history (e.g. "I have gone through many tests and no illness was found"), reflection on personal history (e.g. "I know many people who have belly pain but only one was diagnosed with cancer"), reflections of the treatment history (e.g. "Dr A reviewed my records thoroughly and found no evidence of serious illness"). If a patient struggles, a physician could ask "If your friend struggled with the same worry, what evidence could you give them that would not support the concern?"

As the final, fourth step, both "evidence" supporting and refuting the catastrophic belief should be summarized and consolidated into a single statement. For example, "Although my aunt was diagnosed with cancer, I hear that cancer can be undetected and we have not been able to find the cause of my belly pain, none of my testing so far indicates cancer, most people with belly pain do not have cancer and Dr. A has been thorough in reviewing my records and found no indication of cancer." Patients should be asked to reflect on how they feel when a compound, balanced statement is made.

Typically, bringing together both pro and con "evidence" leads to anxiety decrease. It should be highlighted that all "evidence" is based on the patient's own knowledge and experience. Patients should be asked to practice **cognitive disputation** alone (see Resources for options) or within the context of psychotherapy. It is imperative to remember that **cognitive disputation** is not a technique for outsmarting the patient nor is it a strategy for finding flaws within a patient's beliefs. The goal is to help patients examine their own beliefs and come up with a more balanced view which fully explains their experience. This strategy can reduce both "buy into" catastrophic thoughts and associated distress. For further information about **cognitive disputation**, see Hunter et al. [22] and Beck [9].

2. **Behavioral Avoidance and Safety Behaviors**

Avoidance is a powerful behavioral mechanism which maintains anxiety and distress. Patients suffering from **SSD/IAD** may avoid medical visits, reminders of feared symptoms, and opportunities for social engagement which provide distraction.

Avoidance contributes to **SSD/IAD** primarily via two mechanisms. Firstly, it does not allow the patient to experience the feared stimuli (e.g. event, experience, thought) thus reinforcing belief that the feared stimuli are dangerous. Thus, through avoiding, the patient prevents themselves from learning that feared stimuli is safe or at least not as dangerous as they believe. To illustrate this concept and its consequences, "Feeding the Hungry Tiger" Acceptance and Commitment (ACT) metaphor can be helpful (See Resources) in illustrating both the process and its consequences.

Secondly, **avoidance** acts as a driving force in the process of negative reinforcement. Anxious patient who avoids anxiety triggers/feelings, gradually becomes increasingly reactive to progressively lesser stimuli furthering **avoidance**. This process is known as sensitization. Patients suffering from **SSD/IAD** will often urgently seek medical attention for routine and non-urgent situations. Seeking and receiving urgent reassurance for non-urgent concerns, feeds into the cycle of negative affect/fear **avoidance**.

How to address? It is important to recognize **avoidance** behaviors and negative reinforcement as primary contributors to the patient's distress. Educating the patient about these mechanisms and their consequences can support more effective treatment plans. In the context of ongoing care, the patient and physician may benefit from an explicit agreement about how results, new symptoms, or other emergent concerns will be addressed. Additionally, a list of "red flag" symptoms should be provided with the teach-back utilized to ensure patient's understanding of these symptoms. Patients should be instructed to use **cognitive disputation** and emotional regulation techniques to quell high anxiety.

Reassuringly, **avoidance** can be decreased effectively via non-pharmacological routes. Specifically, a 12-week-long psychotherapy intervention targeting **avoidance** and **safety behaviors** reported clinically significant improvements in health-related anxiety among 53% (therapist-guided internet-based intervention), 48% (self-guided internet-based intervention) and 44% (bibliotherapy intervention) participants. It is noteworthy that participants who engaged in self-paced interventions (electronic or bibliotherapy) demonstrated symptom improvement comparable to those who received therapist's guidance [20].

3. **Difficulties with Strong Negative Emotions and Uncertainty**

Awareness of **negative emotions** (e.g. anxiety, fear, anger) and ability to regulate these emotions is central to wellbeing. **Anxiety sensitivity** (AS) is a psychological characteristic whereby anxiety-related experiences are perceived in catastrophic ways [36]. AS is associated with several SSD/**IAD**-related challenges including greater somatic symptom severity, worse chronic illness control, increased symptom burden, worse functioning and medication nonadherence [1, 15].

How to address? Negative emotions are reciprocally connected with both **catastrophizing** (cognition) and **avoidance** (behaviors) thus mutually reinforcing. Scheduled worry time, also known as Stimulus Control Training, SCT [10] can be effective for sensitizing patients to negative affect.

Stimulus Control Training (SCT)

For SCT practice, patients are asked to schedule daily (same time and same location) 30-min worry time. During SCT practice, patients are encouraged to worry as much as possible. Over time, however, patients can utilize **cognitive disputation** or other techniques to effectively manage their worries. SCT allows for patients to learn that "worry does not pervade their lives throughout the day, and they are able to focus on employing effective coping techniques for their worries in a structured, time-limited setting" [10, p. 194].

Psychothery Effectiveness for SSD/IAD

Overall, meta-analyses of RCTs support the utility of Cognitive Behavioral Therapy (CBT) in treatment of **SSD** and medically unexplained symptoms. Group format was found more effective (−4.43, 95% CI [−8.47, −0.39]) than individual sessions (−1.00, 95% CI [−1.90, −0.10]) in reducing somatic symptoms. Longer course of treatment (i.e. over 12 weeks) and longer duration of each session were found more effective than treatment of shorter duration. [29].

Moreover, brief interventions may be of substantial benefit for **SSD**. Johnson and colleagues (2020) report significant and sustained reduction in **SSD** symptoms following a single, 30-minute session which provided information about "brain pathways for pain and the body's response to stress" while utilizing motivational interviewing techniques and exploring patients' concerns. Specifically, 12.82% reduction in worry was noted following the intervention. Significant reductions were also noted in hospital admissions (d = .36), days admitted to the hospital (d = .47), and inpatient consultations (d = .42).

Unfortunately, both changes in nosology and frequent interchangeable use of terms in research (**SSD**, **IAD**, medically unexplained symptoms, somatic symptom distress, somatoform disorders) limit definitive conclusions from the EBP research. Moreover, some concerns exist around psychotherapists' low comfort with **SSD** diagnosis and treatment (Weigel et al. 2020).

Case Vignette—Continued
Prior to her next visit with Dr. A, Ms. M receives her blood test results indicating iron deficiency anemia. The findings were otherwise normal. Dr. A received several messages to her work inbox, as follows:

Patient's Message #1: *I noticed that some of my bloodwork is highlighted in yellow. I cannot wait until Monday to find out what it all means. Is it cancer?* (**catastrophizing**).

Patient's Message #2: *I already tried calling the front desk, lab, and nurses but I was unable to reach anyone. Please call me back as soon as possible.* (difficulty with strong **negative emotions**/uncertainty).

Dr. A also notes that Ms. M missed several follow-up appointments with her specialists since her last visit (behavioral **avoidance**).

Dr. A calls Ms. M to follow-up:

Dr. A: *Hello Ms. M. I am calling to follow-up with you about the messages you recently sent.*

Ms. M: *Thank you for calling me back! I did not think I was going to hear from you!* (**catastrophizing**) *I have been crying this entire weekend!*

Dr. A: *It is understandable that concerns about your health cause anxiety.*

Ms. M: *I will try anything at this point. I just want to go back to living my life.*

Dr. A: *Next time you feel worried I would like you to try* [Reviews **Cognitive Disputation** for **Catastrophizing**]. What do you think about this plan?

Ms. M: *I think this is a good start to help me focus less on my negative thoughts and more on all the reasons why I might not be seriously ill.*

Dr. A: *I also wanted to talk about what to do when new or more severe symptoms come up. Perhaps we can come up with a list of dangerous signs that you can look at before considering medical attention.*

Ms. M: *This would be helpful because otherwise I either feel like I need to call someone or go to the ED.*

Dr. A: [Dr. A reviews 'Red Flag' symptoms] *If you notice that none of the symptoms are in the dangerous category, we can plan to meet in 6 weeks to discuss these. To make sure that I clearly explained the plan, can you please tell me what our plan is, moving forward?*

Ms. M: *When I get anxious about my stomach pain or feel like something terrible might happen, I will make a list with things that support and don't support my worry. I will then make one statement to balance all of them.*

Dr. A: *Exactly. What about if you feel like you need to speak to someone right away about your symptoms or a blood test?*

Ms. M: *I will review the list you sent me with the scary symptoms. If I do not have any of those, we can meet at my next appointment in 6 weeks.*

Integrative Medicine Interventions and Techniques

A range of **mind-body** practices (MBPs) can cultivate non-judgmental self-awareness and promote regulation of the hyperarousal symptoms associated with **SSD/IAD** [37]. MBPs include mindfulness-based stress reduction (MBSR), yoga, meditation, guided imagery, biofeedback, and breathwork. Overarchingly, these approaches support reappraisal of stressful events and physical experiences thus leading to improved emotional regulation [17]. Furthermore, meta-analytic findings report that mindfulness-based psychotherapeutic interventions are "promising" for treatment of SSD/**IAD** [30].

This section overviews initial steps to introducing MBPs to the patient. Selection of the specific technique is contingent on patient's preference, physician's competence/training and access/availability factors. Effective implementation of MBPs requires a collaborative patient-physician relationship to navigate distress associated with waxing and waning trajectory of physical symptoms that characterize **SSD/IAD.**

To introduce mindfulness techniques, clinicians can use the following inquiry:

1. Explore the patient's pre-existing notions of the **mind-body** connection: "*What is your understanding of the brain/mind and body connection as it relates to your symptoms?*"
2. Ask for permission to offer education around **mind-body** connection that is specific to the patients' symptoms "*Is it ok if I share some information about how your brain and mind are intimately connected to your physical symptoms?*"
3. Use accessible visuals (e.g., pictures or videos) to provide education on the **mind-body** connection during the visit. Patients can also independently review educational materials following/between visits. The education material should relate to the patients' physical symptoms as demonstrated in the examples below:
   (a) For a patient with palpitations, show a diagram of the sympathetic and parasympathetic nervous system with innervation to the heart: "*Stressful thoughts can activate the sympathetic nervous system. This is how your body will respond if you were chased by a wild animal. When sympathetic nervous system is active it turns on the body's "fight or flight" mode leading to increased heart rate and palpitations.*
   (b) For a patient with gastrointestinal symptoms, show an image of the "gut-brain" axis: "*The gastrointestinal system and the brain are intimately connected through several mechanisms including the vagus nerve, microbiome, and chemicals that communicate through the blood stream.*"
4. Introduce the concept of MBPs: "*Mind–body practices are techniques that can help your body and mind work together to improve your symptoms.*"
5. Individualize the **mind-body** intervention: "*Can I tell you more about the types of* ***mind-body*** *techniques that have been shown to be helpful for your symptoms, and you can choose which one you'd like to explore?*"

Please see the Resources section for mindfulness practice resources.

Clinical Pearls

- **SSD/IAD** diagnosis should focus on a patient's excessive distress related to the somatic symptoms (or possibility of developing a medical condition). Whether symptoms are/are not medically explained is not pertinent to these diagnoses.
- Introduce biopsychosocial conceptualization at the start of the treatment, noting relevance of both mind and body in the illness course and management.
- Discuss limitations of medical testing and procedures—these are unlikely to assuage concerns for patients with **SSD/IAD**.

- Address symptom **catastrophizing** while helping the patients understand symptoms which require care escalation ("red flags").
- Be mindful about the role of **avoidance,** particularly the role of seeking care in the process of negative reinforcement.
- Communicate empathy for patients' experience while helping to build skills in tolerating **negative emotions.**

Frequently Asked Questions

Question 1: *This* [physical symptoms] *cannot just be in my head, what is causing my symptoms?*

Answer: Your physical symptoms cause you bodily discomfort but also make you very worried. This worry is likely making physical symptoms feel even worse. When you try to avoid unpleasant situations or interpret events catastrophically, anxiety is likely to worsen. Let's make sure that we are managing your health-related worries and coping strategies.

Question 2: *Can't you just give me something to make [symptoms] go away*?

Answer: Unfortunately, your symptoms are long-term and there may not be a perfect medication to get rid of them completely. Good news is that you can take several steps to improve both your symptoms and your quality of life. These involve both medication and non-medication options as both are important to optimizing health.

Question 3: *I googled my symptoms and then also asked ChatGPT about them and now I am really freaked out. What should I do?*

Answer: Googling, using ChatGPT, or otherwise researching symptoms online, often does not help to resolve medical concerns. If you have questions about your physical symptoms, please write these down before our next meeting and we can review these together so that I can address your concerns.

Case Vignette—Conclusion

Four weeks after the diagnosis of **SSD**, Ms. M is back in the office to see Dr. A:

Dr. A: *How are you feeling since we last spoke?*

Ms. M: *Sometimes I feel like I just spend the entire day worrying about my symptoms. It feels like I cannot get anything done.*

Dr. A: *There is a technique that we can talk about to help decrease the amount of time you spend worrying* [Reviews Stimulus Control Training].

Ms. M: *If I can get down to worrying just 30 min out of my day, that would free me up to do so much! I feel bad because I spent so much time worrying that I just couldn't make it to those specialist appointments.*

Dr. A: *At times, anxiety may cause us to avoid things that may be important for us to do. In the long run, this may lead us to actions that can increase distress.* [Reviews Behavioral **Avoidance** and **Safety Behaviors**].

Ms. M: *I want to get better, but I need help getting out of my head.*

Dr. A: *There are multiple strategies to accomplish your goals. These can involve self-help options or possible referrals for mental health support to address your symptoms. Let's discuss the plan which works best for you.*

Resources

Source	Description	Link
Braive—Youtube Channel	Video outlines the effect of stress upon health and supports a holistic view of mind/body Duration 2:25	https://www.youtube.com/watch?v=Ba_A43kzNBw
Cleavland clinic	Brief, patient focused description of SSD, causes, and treatment options	Somatic Symptom Disorder: What It Is, Symptoms & Treatment
Hayes, S.C., & Smith, S. (2005). Get out of your mind and into your life. The new Acceptance and Commitment Therapy. New Harbinger Publications. pp 36–37.	Tiger Metaphor outlines process of avoidance and its consequences	https://contextualscience.org/sites/default/files/ACT%20FOR%20LIFE%20ANXIETYACBS.pdf
Nathan, P., Rees, C., Lim, L., & Correia, H. (2003). Back from the Bluez. Perth, Western Australia: Centre for Clinical Interventions Module 6: Detective Work and Disputation	Patient handout assisting with cognitive disputation task	Module 6: Detective Work and Disputation
Palouse Mindfulness. (n.d.). *Palouse Mindfulness: Free online MBSR training*. https://palousemindfulness.com/index.html	Free online online Mindfulness-Based Stress Reduction (MBSR) course	https://palousemindfulness.com/index.html
Arizona State University, T. Denny Sanford School of Social and Family Dynamics.	Multiple mindfulness scripts including: breath awareness, belly breathing, guided imagery, body scan etc.	https://thesanfordschool.asu.edu/sites/g/files/litvpz486/files/2022-07/Mindfulness%20Scripts_Combined.pdf

References

1. Alcántara C, Qian M, Meli L, Ensari I, Ye S, Davidson KW, Diaz KM. Anxiety sensitivity and physical inactivity in a national sample of adults with a history of myocardial infarction. Int J Behav Med. 2020;27(5):520–6. https://doi.org/10.1007/s12529-020-09881-w.
2. AlHadi AN, AlAteeq DA, Al-Sharif E, Bawazeer HM, Alanazi H, AlShomrani AT, Shuqdar RM, AlOwaybil R. An Arabic translation, reliability, and validation of patient health questionnaire in a Saudi sample. Ann Gen Psychiatry. 2017;16:32. https://doi.org/10.1186/s12991-017-0155-1.

3. Alshayea AK. Latent structure, measurement invariance, and reliability of an Arabic version of the short health anxiety inventory. J Exp Psychopathol. 2020;11(2):1–15. https://doi.org/10.1177/2043808720912629.
4. American Psychiatric Association. Diagnostic and statistical manual of mental disorders (5th ed., text revised). Arlington: Author; 2022.
5. American Psychiatric Association, Division of Research. Highlights of changes from DSM-IV to DSM-5: somatic symptom and related disorders. Focus. 2013;11(4):525–7. Retrieved from https://psychiatryonline.org/doi/full/10.1176/appi.focus.11.4.525.
6. Arnáez S, García-Soriano G, López-Santiago J, Belloch A. The Spanish validation of the short health anxiety inventory: psychometric properties and clinical utility. Int J Clin Health Psychol. 2019;19(3):251–60. https://doi.org/10.1016/j.ijchp.2019.05.003.
7. Barbek RME, Makowski AC, von dem Knesebeck O. Social inequalities in health anxiety: A systematic review and meta-analysis. J Psychosom Res. 2022;153:110706. https://doi-org.ezproxy.cul.columbia.edu/10.1016/j.jpsychores.2021.110706.
8. Barbek R, Toussaint A, Löwe B, et al. Intersectional inequalities in somatic symptom severity in the adult population in Germany found within the SOMA.SOC study. Sci Rep. 2024;14:3820. https://doi.org/10.1038/s41598-024-54042-8.
9. Beck, J. (2021). Cognitive behavior therapy. Basics and beyond. 3rd Ed. Guildford Press, New York.
10. Behar E, Borkovec TD. Avoiding treatment failures in generalized anxiety disorder. In: Otto MW, Hofmann S, editors. Avoiding treatment failures in the anxiety disorders. New York: Springer; 2009. p. 185–208.
11. Creed F. The predictors of somatic symptoms in a population sample: the lifelines cohort study. Psychosom Med. 2022;84(9):1056–66. https://doi.org/10.1097/PSY.0000000000001101.
12. de Vroege L, Hoedeman R, Nuyen J, Sijtsma K, van der Feltz-Cornelis CM. Validation of the PHQ-15 for somatoform disorder in the occupational health care setting. J Occup Rehabil. 2012;22(1):51–8. https://doi.org/10.1007/s10926-011-9320-6.
13. Dimsdale JE, Creed F, Escobar J, Sharpe M, Wulsin L, Barsky A, Lee S, Irwin MR, Levenson J. Somatic symptom disorder: an important change in DSM. J Psychosom Res. 2013;75(3):223–8. https://doi-org.ezproxy.cul.columbia.edu/10.1016/j.jpsychores.2013.06.033.
14. Duclos A, Frits ML, Iannaccone C, Lipsitz SR, Cooper Z, Weissman JS, et al. Safety of inpatient care in surgical settings: cohort study. BMJ. 2024;387:e080480. https://doi.org/10.1136/bmj-2024-080480.
15. Favreau H, Bacon SL, Labrecque M, Lavoie KL. Prospective impact of panic disorder and panic-anxiety on asthma control, health service use, and quality of life in adult patients with asthma over a 4-year follow-up. Psychosom Med. 2014;76(2):147–55. https://doi.org/10.1097/PSY.0000000000000032.
16. Fink P, Ewald H, Jensen J, Sørensen L, Engberg M, Holm M, Munk-Jørgensen P. Screening for somatization and hypochondriasis in primary care and neurological in-patients: a seven-item scale for hypochondriasis and somatization. J Psychosom Res. 1999;46(3):261–73. https://doi.org/10.1016/s0022-3999(98)00092-0.
17. Garland EL, Hanley A, Farb NA, Froeliger BE. State mindfulness during meditation predicts enhanced cognitive reappraisal. Mindfulness. 2015;6(2):234–42. https://doi.org/10.1007/s12671-013-0250-6.
18. Gierk B, Kohlmann S, Kroenke K, Spangenberg L, Zenger M, Brähler E, Löwe B. The somatic symptom scale-8 (SSS-8): a brief measure of somatic symptom burden. JAMA Intern Med. 2014;174(3):399–407. https://doi.org/10.1001/jamainternmed.2013.12179.
19. Han C, Pae CU, Patkar AA, Masand PS, Kim KW, Joe SH, Jung IK. Psychometric properties of the Patient Health Questionnaire-15 (PHQ-15) for measuring the somatic symptoms of psychiatric outpatients. Psychosomatics. 2009;50(6):580–5. https://doi-org.ezproxy.cul.columbia.edu/10.1176/appi.psy.50.6.580.

20. Hedman E, Axelsson E, Andersson E, Lekander M, Ljótsson B. Exposure-based cognitive-behavioural therapy via the internet and as bibliotherapy for somatic symptom disorder and illness anxiety disorder: randomised controlled trial. Br J Psychiatry J Ment Sci. 2016;209(5):407–13. https://doi-org.ezproxy.cul.columbia.edu/10.1192/bjp.bp.116.181396.
21. Hennemann S, Böhme K, Kleinstäuber M, Baumeister H, Küchler AM, Ebert DD, Witthöft M. Internet-based CBT for somatic symptom distress (iSOMA) in emerging adults: A randomized controlled trial. J Consult Clin Psychol. 2022;90(4):353–65. https://doi-org.ezproxy.cul.columbia.edu/10.1037/ccp0000707.
22. Hunter CL, Goodie JL, Oordt MS, Dobmeyer AC. Integrated behavioral health in primary care: Step-by-step guidance for assessment and intervention (2nd ed.). American Psychological Association. 2017. https://doi-org.ezproxy.cul.columbia.edu/10.1037/0000017-000.
23. Johnson KK, Bennett C, Rochani H. Significant improvement of somatic symptom disorder with brief psychoeducational intervention by PMHNP in primary care. J Am Psychiatr Nurses Assoc. 2022;28(2):171–80. https://doi-org.ezproxy.cul.columbia.edu/10.1177/1078390320960524.
24. Kabat-Zinn J. An outpatient program in behavioral medicine for chronic pain patients based on the practice of mindfulness meditation: theoretical considerations and preliminary results. Gen Hosp Psychiatry. 1982;4(1):33–47. https://doi.org/10.1016/0163-8343(82)90026-3.
25. Khalil H, Huang C. Adverse drug reactions in primary care: a scoping review. BMC Health Serv Res. 2020;20(1):5. https://doi.org/10.1186/s12913-019-4651-7.
26. Khan AA, Khan A, Harezlak J, Tu W, Kroenke K. Somatic symptoms in primary care: etiology and outcome. Psychosomatics. 2003;44(6):471–8. https://doi-org.ezproxy.cul.columbia.edu/10.1176/appi.psy.44.6.471
27. Kroenke K, Spitzer RL, Williams JB. The PHQ-15: validity of a new measure for evaluating the severity of somatic symptoms. Psychosom Med. 2002;64(2):258–66. https://doi.org/10.1097/00006842-200203000-00008.
28. Li T, Wei J, Fritzsche K, Toussaint AC, Zhang L, Zhang Y, Chen H, Wu H, Ma X, Li W, Ren J, Lu W, Leonhart R. Validation of the Chinese version of the somatic symptom Scale-8 in patients from tertiary hospitals in China. Front Psych. 2022;13:940206. https://doi.org/10.3389/fpsyt.2022.940206.
29. Liu J, Gill NS, Teodorczuk A, Li ZJ, Sun J. The efficacy of cognitive behavioural therapy in somatoform disorders and medically unexplained physical symptoms: A meta-analysis of randomized controlled trials. J Affect Disord. 2019;245:98–112. https://doi-org.ezproxy.cul.columbia.edu/10.1016/j.jad.2018.10.114.
30. Maas Genannt Bermpohl F, Hülsmann L, Martin A. Efficacy of mindfulness- and acceptance-based cognitive-behavioral therapies for bodily distress in adults: a meta-analysis. Front Psych. 2023;14:1160908. https://doi.org/10.3389/fpsyt.2023.1160908.
31. Murray AM, Toussaint A, Althaus A, Löwe B. The challenge of diagnosing non-specific, functional, and somatoform disorders: A systematic review of barriers to diagnosis in primary care. J Psychosom Res. 2016;80:1-10 https://doi.org/10.1016/j.jpsychores.2015.11.002.
32. NovoPsych. Short Health Anxiety Inventory (SHAI). n.d. Retrieved September 30, 2025 from https://novopsych.com/assessments/health/short-health-anxiety-inventory-shai/.
33. Pan X, Ding W, Sun X, Ji C, Zhou Q, Yan C, Zhou Y, Luo Y. Gray matter density of the dorsomedial prefrontal cortex mediates the relationship between catastrophizing and anxiety in somatic symptom disorder. Neuropsychiatr Dis Treat. 2021;17:757–64. https://doi-org.ezproxy.cul.columbia.edu/10.2147/NDT.S29646.
34. Pfizer. Welcome to the Patient Health Questionnaire (PHQ) Screeners. Screener overview. n.d. Retrieved from: https://www.phqscreeners.com/select-screener
35. Pilipenko N. Somatic symptom disorder in primary care: a collaborative approach. J Fam Pract. 2022;71(3):E8–E12. https://doi-org.ezproxy.cul.columbia.edu/10.12788/jfp.0384.
36. Reiss S, Peterson RA, Gursky DM, McNally RJ. Anxiety sensitivity, anxiety frequency and the prediction of fearfulness. Behav Res Ther. 1986;24(1):1–8. https://doi.org/10.1016/0005-7967(86)90143-9.

37. Ring M, Mahadevan R. Introduction to integrative medicine in the primary care setting. Prim Care. 2017;44(2):203–15. https://doi.org/10.1016/j.pop.2017.02.006.
38. Robles E, Angelone C, Ondé D, Vázquez C. Somatic symptoms in the general population of Spain: validation and normative data of the patient health Questionnaire-15 (PHQ-15). J Affect Disord. 2024;362:762–71. https://doi.org/10.1016/j.jad.2024.07.087.
39. Salkovskis PM, Rimes KA, Warwick HMC, Clark DM. The health anxiety inventory: development and validation of scales for the measurement of health anxiety and hypochondriasis. Psychol Med. 2002;32(5):843–53. https://doi.org/10.1017/S0033291702005822.
40. van Ravesteijn H, Wittkampf K, Lucassen P, van de Lisdonk E, van den Hoogen H, van Weert H, Huijser J, Schene A, van Weel C, Speckens A. Detecting somatoform disorders in primary care with the PHQ-15. Ann Fam Med. 2009;7(3):232–8. https://doi-org.ezproxy.cul.columbia.edu/10.1370/afm.985.
41. Verdurmen MJ, Videler AC, Kamperman AM, Khasho D, van der Feltz-Cornelis CM. Cognitive behavioral therapy for somatic symptom disorders in later life: a prospective comparative explorative pilot study in two clinical populations. Neuropsychiatr Dis Treat. 2017;13:2331–9. https://doi-org.ezproxy.cul.columbia.edu/10.2147/NDT.S141208.
42. Verhaak PF, Meijer SA, Visser AP, Wolters G. Persistent presentation of medically unexplained symptoms in general practice. Fam Pract. 2006;23(4):414–20. https://doi-org.ezproxy.cul.columbia.edu/10.1093/fampra/cml016
43. Zhang Y, Liu R, Li G, Mao S, Yuan Y. The reliability and validity of a Chinese-version short health anxiety inventory: an investigation of university students. Neuropsychiatr Dis Treat. 2015;11:1739–47. https://doi.org/10.2147/NDT.S83501.
44. Zhang L, Fritzsche K, Liu Y, Wang J, Huang M, Wang Y, Chen L, Luo S, Yu J, Dong Z, Mo L, Leonhart R. Validation of the Chinese version of the PHQ-15 in a tertiary hospital. BMC Psychiatry. 2016;16:89. https://doi.org/10.1186/s12888-016-0798-5.

Chapter 3
Panic Disorder

Nataliya Pilipenko, Krishna M. Desai, and Aury Garcia

Case Vignette: Part 1

Mr. V is a 55-year-old man with a history of chronic kidney disease and diabetes who is presenting for evaluation of palpitations.

Mr. V: *For the last two months, I get these episodes when my heart is racing. When this happens, I cannot breathe, my chest starts to hurt, and both of my hands start to tingle. I get really scared. I went to the ED a few times because I thought I might be dying.*

Dr. L: *Scary symptoms! You said you went to the ED too. What did the doctors there tell you?*

Mr. V: *I have been to the ED but also saw a heart doctor. They checked my blood, did an EKG, chest x-ray, an ultrasound of my heart, and even checked for an abnormal heartbeat but could not find anything.*

Dr. L: *Is there anything specific that triggers these symptoms?*

N. Pilipenko (✉)
Center for Family and Community Medicine, Department of Medicine, Columbia University Irving Medical Center/New York Presbyterian Hospital, New York, NY, USA

Department of Psychiatry, Columbia University Irving Medical Center, New York, NY, USA
e-mail: np2615@cumc.columbia.edu

K. M. Desai
Center for Family and Community Medicine, Department of Medicine, Columbia University Irving Medical Center/New York Presbyterian Hospital, New York, NY, USA

Center for Neuroinflammatory and Somatic Disorders, Department of Psychiatry, Columbia University Irving Medical Center, New York, NY, USA

A. Garcia
Center for Family and Community Medicine, Department of Medicine, Columbia University Irving Medical Center/New York Presbyterian Hospital, New York, NY, USA

N. Pilipenko, K. M. Desai (eds.), *8 Conditions Primary Care Clinicians Dread to Treat*, https://doi.org/10.1007/978-3-032-12819-5_3

Mr. V: *No idea. They happen randomly at all hours of the day at least once per week. I even stopped drinking coffee to see if these symptoms would go away, but no luck. I just can't figure out why [symptoms are happening]. I smoked cigarettes but quit 15 years ago. I only drink a glass of wine every month or two for a special occasion. I don't use drugs, just take my diabetes medication.*

Dr. L: *Can you tell me a bit more about how the symptoms you described affect your daily life?*

Mr. V: *Over the last month, I constantly worry that it might happen again. I feel like I cannot leave my apartment to see my friends and family or do my errands, just in case something happens to bring on one of the episodes. No luck though, I can be watching tv, or showering, or just doing nothing when it hits me.*

Dr. L: *Let's work together to figure out what is going on and create a plan to better manage your symptoms.*

Diagnosis: Brief Description

Per DSM-5-TR [3], **PD** is defined by presence of recurrent **panic attack**s (**PA**s), at least some of which occur "out of the blue." To meet diagnostic criteria, at least four of the following thirteen symptoms should be present during a **PA**: palpitations, sweating, trembling/shaking, subjective sensation of being short of breath and/or smothering, choking, chest pain/discomfort, nausea or gastrointestinal distress, dizziness/unsteadiness/light-headedness, chills or heat sensations, paresthesias, derealization/depersonalization, fear of loss of control/going crazy, fear of dying [3, pp. 235–236].

Although **PA**s may occur within the context of any psychiatric disorder, distinguishing feature of the **PD** is either ongoing worry about **PA** recurrence (for at least 1 month) and/or "significant maladaptive changes in behavior" (3, p. 236) aimed at reducing possibility of future attacks. Avoidance behaviors may also focus on efforts to minimize **interoceptive** sensations (i.e. sensations about the body's internal state) which resemble **PA** symptoms. For example, patients may reduce caffeine intake, physical activities or exposure to specific events (e.g., watching scary films, interpersonal conflicts, sexual activities) as these increase sympathetic arousal resembling **PA** symptoms.

Physicians should be mindful that substances (including heavy metals or toxins), medication or drugs (e.g., cannabis, caffeine, stimulants, bronchodilators, anticholinergics, corticosteroids, lithium, anticonvulsants etc.), and medical conditions (e.g. hyperthyroidism, hypoglycemia, congestive heart failure, arrhythmias, chronic obstructive pulmonary disease, vitamin B12 deficiency, seizure disorders) are ruled out when **PD** is suspected. Please refer to DSM-5-TR [3] for information pertaining to the differential diagnostic considerations.

Prevalence, Risk Factors, and Disparities

Among the U.S. general population, lifetime prevalence of isolated **PA**s is 22.7% [15]. However, lifetime prevalence of **PD** is 4.7% [12] and 12-month prevalence is estimated at 2–3% [3, p. 237]. Thus, while **PA**s are common, only a fraction of persons who experience a **PA** go on to develop **PD**. Moreover, approximately a half of patients receiving **PD** treatment report prodromal panic-like sensations before their first **PA** [9].

In the U.S., significantly higher rates of **PD** are noted among non-Latinx Whites as compared to Latinx, African American, Caribbean Blacks, and Asian Americans. Within the non-Latinx White group, females are twice as likely to endorse **PD** as males [3, p. 237]. Limited research suggests that specific of **PD** symptom reporting can differ across ethnic groups [5]. However, when suspecting **PD** physicians need to be aware of culturally bound concepts of distress which can resemble **panic attack**s, such as ataque de nervios and khyal cap (see [3, pp. 874–875] for further discussion).

PD risk factors include chronic stress, parental overprotection and low emotional warmth, poor access to economic resources, family history of **PD**, tobacco use, and medical conditions affecting the respiratory system [3, pp. 238–239].

Symptom Assessment Tools

Table 3.1 presents three common **PD** screening tools. Patient Health Questionnaire for **Panic Disorder** (PHQ-**PD**) [26] and **Panic Disorder** Screener [4, 6] assess symptoms in the prior four weeks (per DSM-5-TR criteria) while **Panic Disorder** Severity Scale (PDSS) [25] uses a shorter timeline (one week). PHQ-**PD** is the only screening tool which makes inquiries about specific **PA** symptoms while PADIS and PDSS present the symptoms and ask patients to complete questions on avoidance and distress if four or more of **PA** symptoms are present. Finally, PHQ-**PD** assesses only **PA**-related distress/worry but not **PA**-related avoidance.

Table 3.1 Panic disorder screening tools

Screener name	Items #	Rating scale scoring	Cut offs	Assessment timeline	Availability	Psychometric properties	Non-english versions available?
Patient Health Questionnaire for Panic Disorder (PHQ-PD)	15 [26]	Binary [26] 0 = No 1 = Yes	PHQ-PD [26] consists of 2 sections, 4 items establishing PD symptoms, followed by 11 items assessing PA symptoms For positive screening score, patient endorse all 4 PD items and at least 4 of PA items [26]	4 week [26]	Open access [22]	Sensitivity = .81 [26] Specificity = .99 Validation in Spanish [20] reported sensitivity = .83 associated with 1st item of PHQ-PD "In the last 4 weeks, have you had an anxiety attack — suddenly feeling fear or panic?"	Arabic [1], Chinese [22], Spanish [22]
Panic Disorder Screener (PADIS)	4 [6]	Item 1: 5-point likert [6] Items 2–4: 4-point likert Item 1: 0 = none to 4 = more than 11 panic episodes Items 2–4: 0 = never to 3 = all the time	Score ≥4 [6], Sensitivity = .77 Specificity = .84	1 month [6]	Open access [4]	Good internal consistency (Cronbach α = .86) [6] Every 1-point increase in PADIS score is associated with 69% increased odds of meeting clinical criteria for PD	None

Panic Disorder Severity Scale (PDSS)	7 [21]	5-point Likert [21] 0 = no/not at [21] all/none to 4 = extreme/ extremely/nearly constantly Raw scores range 0–28	Score of ≥9 [21] suggests a need for formal diagnostic assessment for PD	4 week [21]	Open access [21]	Original internal consistency (α = .64) [25] Follow-up studies showing good internal consistency (Cronbach α = .83 for clinician administered and α = .80 for patient self-report) [27]	Chinese [18], Spanish [10]

Non-pharmacological Conceptualization: What to Say to the Patient?

Effective care of **PD** requires effective communication about its etiology and maintaining factors. Three messages below outline specifics.

Message #1: Fight-Flight-Freeze (FFF) Response Underlies Panic Attacks

Built to protect from danger, **FFF** automatically "turns on" in a dangerous situation. **FFF** manifests via **PA** symptoms such as rapid heart rate, sweating, trembling, muscle tension, tunnel vision etc. All these physical symptoms mobilize the body for survival. Unfortunately, the human brain does not differentiate between anxiety and danger. When encountering a threat (e.g., deadlines, bills, medical tests) it only has **FFF** as a response and turns it on quickly. While **PA**s are frightening, these are not dangerous and do not cause harm. It is our body's well intentioned, although misguided, attempt to defend against something frightening.

Why? It is imperative for patients to understand the underlying mechanism behind the **PA**s. This knowledge can normalize the experience, reduce anxiety and promote treatment engagement. Explanation both de-pathologized and de-catastrophizes **PA**s which are subjectively extremely frightening. Please see the Resources section for sample metaphors/analogies used to describe **PA** and **FFF** as well as patient education resources.

Message #2: In PD, PAs May Not Be Triggered by Fear or Stress

While **PA**s can be triggered by worries or stress, they can also frequently happen because **FFF** "turned on" without apparent threat or danger. In fact, **PD** diagnosis requires that some of the **PA**s happen "out of the blue". This is the result of the **FFF** response being both automatic/unconscious and very sensitive. This is an important feature of **FFF** because in life-or-death situations delayed response (even to subtle danger cues) can result in serious harm.

Furthermore, human bodies can read (and misread) their own cues such as changes in breathing, fear-related thoughts, and feelings. Internal physical sensations (also known as **interoceptive** sensations) such as increases in heart rate (after drinking coffee), shakiness (after drinking alcohol), sweating (when being in hot rooms) can serve as reminders of **PA** symptoms. When physical sensations are noticed, they are perceived as frightening (e.g. What if my shortness of breath is a sign of a heart attack?) leading to **FFF** activation.

Why? Patients experiencing **PA**s within the context of **PD** often do not experience triggering stressful events. Thus, explanations which focus on anxiety/stress/fear are not seen as relevant by the patient. It is essential to be aware of the "out of the blue" nature of **PA**s within **PD** and introduce **FFF** concept as soon as possible to reduce associated anxiety and unnecessary use of medical services.

Message #3: Avoidance of PA Leads to More PAs

Many patients (reasonably) respond to **PA**s by trying to reduce their recurrence by avoiding situations or experiences which may lead to **PA**s. Although this behavior is logical, it leads to a paradoxical increase in frequency and severity of **PA**s and consequent distress and functional impairment. **PD** presentation is unique as symptoms come from catastrophic perceptions of own physical sensations, not a real danger. So, to treat **PA**s effectively, what needs to be changed are perceptions of symptoms.

Why? Avoidance functions as a primary mechanism of **PA** recurrence and exacerbation. When avoiding possible **PA**s (this can be via non-engagement or using safety behaviors), patients are unable to learn that symptoms are transient and do not lead to feared consequences. Furthermore, avoidance leads to sensitization, a process by which the patient will become progressively more sensitive to danger cues and **interoceptive** sensations. This sets up a vicious cycle of **PD**.

Case Vignette—Continued
Mr. V returns to see Dr. L about his diagnosis and next steps. He completed the PHQ-**PD** with a score positive for **PD.**

Dr. L: *I was hoping to start by going over my thoughts about your diagnosis with you. Would that be ok?*

Mr. V: *Sure! I have had more of my episodes since I saw you. I have not been going out much. Just try to keep an ice bucket nearby. When I feel it coming on, I stick my hands in. That seems to help.*

Dr. L: *Sounds like you are still struggling with these episodes. Let me share my thoughts with you. [Mr V nods] I reviewed your history, labs, and imaging studies. Your physical exams with me and in the past are all normal. Your score on the questionnaire that you completed earlier today, confirms my suspicion that [symptoms] are likely due to a condition called panic disorder. Have you heard anything about it?*

Mr. V: *No, I have not.*

Dr. L: Can I tell you about this diagnosis?

Mr. V: Please do!

Dr. L: [Discusses Message #1 and #2]. *What questions do you have for me about **PD**?*

Mr. V: *No questions. It sounds like I should just stay home, stay relaxed and these will go away, right? My body will calm down.*

Dr. L: *Unfortunately, staying at home is likely to make your symptoms worse.* [Discusses Message #3].

Mr. V: So, what should I do then?

Dr. L: *Like with any condition, it is important to make sure that you become knowledgeable about it, so that you can learn best coping strategies. Also, it's important to know that while* ***PA****s are very scary, they are not dangerous. I would suggest doing two things. First, since you have not heard about* ***PD****, I will give you some materials to read about it. Knowing what is happening can help to make these episodes less scary. Secondly, let's discuss "red flag" symptoms which are likely not due to* ***PD*** *so that if you notice these, you can seek medical attention.*

Non-pharmacological Treatment Options: What Can Be Done?

Patients are often confused about mechanisms of **PD** and/or wish to eliminate symptoms quickly. However, unfortunately the desire to avoid symptoms leads to symptom maintenance and/or exacerbation. This section outlines techniques which can improve **PD** coping and its symptoms.

Normalization and Education

Providing clear education about **PD** is necessary to normalize symptoms and facilitate illness coping. Messages 1–3 articulate main educational points. Additionally, informing patients about **PA** and **PD** prevalence rates and unique symptom profile (especially "out of the blue" rather than stressor-triggered **PA**s within the context of **PD**) can both de-mystify and de-catastrophize **PD**.

Furthermore, patients may benefit from knowledge related to etiological factors. Specifically, **PD** is associated with higher sensitivity to bodily cues and sensations (e.g. changes in breathing, temperature, vestibular changes) and tendency to worry about physical symptoms and meaning of anxiety (also known as "anxiety sensitivity"). Therefore, as part of **PD**, **PA**s may be triggered by subtle changes to the body (e.g. breathing, temperature etc.). Since physical changes tend to be unpredictable and patients with **PD** tend to focus on these sensations, a self-perpetuating cycle of hyperfocus and panic is set up. Unfortunately, however, in **PD** the actual worry about more **PA**s acts as a trigger for the **PA**s (adapted from [9]). It is important to note that **PD** treatments will not aim to eliminate **PA**s (as most patients wish) as **FFF** is physiologically "built in." However, treatments will reduce **PA**-related distress and improve functioning.

Building Coping Skills While Targeting Avoidance

PD is largely maintained by avoidance of both possible and potential **PA** triggers. While leading to short term anxiety reduction, avoidance maintains and worsens **PD** symptoms over time as the patient is unable to learn that **PA** symptoms are not dangerous and will quickly subside unless fueled by catastrophic interpretations of associated physical sensations. Avoidance can become a highly sophisticated behavior and include safety signals (e.g. always carrying anxiolytic medications, remaining close to certain people or places which became associated with safety) or safety behaviors (e.g. avoiding caffeine, strong emotions/excitement, sports). Unfortunately, avoidance behaviors can be unintentionally reinforced by physicians (e.g. "We always want you to come in if you are feeling worried about any symptoms!"). Anxiolytic interventions, such as medications and relaxation techniques should be used judiciously to ensure that avoidance is not strengthened and subsequent suffering and impairment is not prolonged. So, what can be done?

Strategy A. Diaphragmatic Breathing

Breathing skills are incorporated within evidence-based psychotherapy protocols for **PD** (see [9, pp. 85–97]). **Diaphragmatic breathing** is a technique that teaches the patient to deactivate **FFF** and facilitate coping via increased self-efficacy. Patients should be instructed to initially practice **diaphragmatic breathing** for 5 min daily and begin using during **PA**s only when technique is well learned, to avoid hyperventilation which can be associated with over breathing. It is important to emphasize that **diaphragmatic breathing** as a technique for **PD** management, not a panacea to avoid any **PA**-like symptoms.

Strategy B. Emotional Acceptance

Patients with **PD** struggle with inherent paradox: their efforts to keep **PA**s at bay, lead to increased symptoms focus, distress, and catastrophizing, cumulatively resulting in bringing on **PA**s. Hayes and Smith [13], describe this experience as "If you are not willing to have it, you will." (Hayes and Smith [13], p. 30). To counter this tendency, "Unwanted Party Guest" metaphor can be used. In this metaphor, the patient experiences multiple experiences and emotions (i.e. party "guests") some of which can be "unwanted: (e.g. fear, distress). However, excessive focus on the "unwanted guest" does not result in them leaving, only distracts from being able to stay present to enjoy the "party." (See Resources for link to Unwanted Party Guest video).

Combination of education, **diaphragmatic breathing** and acceptance-based techniques lay the foundation for psychotherapy interventions. Patients experiencing **PD** can significantly benefit from applying cognitive disputation technique (See Chapter 2) to examine their beliefs about **PD** symptoms.

Psychotherapy Effectiveness for Panic Disorder (PD)

APA's Society of Clinical Psychology lists cognitive behavioral therapy (CBT) as the only strongly supported EBP for **PD**. While both applied relaxation and psychoanalytic treatments have received research attention, there is limited support for these approaches. With regards to the CBT's effectiveness for **PD**, a systematic review and component network meta-analysis [23] note odds ratio for the remission of 7.69 (95% CI [1.75, 33.33]) associated with CBT. Moreover, prospective cohort study of group-delivered CBT for **PD** [8], notes that 98% of participants reported sustained symptom reduction of 50% after 3 years of treatment completion. Moreover, 95% reported high to very high satisfaction and 93% reported large treatment benefits.

Pompoli and colleagues [23] note that CBT's effectiveness for **PD** is associated with face-to-face and **interoceptive** exposure components but recommend excluding muscle relaxation and virtual-reality exposure techniques as these components are not associated with symptom improvements.

Integrative Medicine Interventions and Techniques

Lifestyle Medicine (LM): Aerobic Activity

Both aerobic and non-aerobic exercise can reduce symptoms of **PD** [14]. More specifically, Gaudlitz et al. [11] report that addition of aerobic exercise moderately enhances outcomes of CBT ($\eta(2)$ p = .072) with results maintained at 7 month follow up.

Mind-Body Techniques: Yoga and Mindfulness Based Interventions (MBIs)

MBIs involve the practice of nonjudgmentally and purposefully paying attention to the moment-by-moment awareness of thoughts, feelings, bodily sensations, and surrounding environment. There are formal (breathing exercises, yoga, mindfulness meditation) and informal practices both of which have potential to improve anxiety symptoms [29].

More specifically, yoga may be valuable to augmentation of PD treatment. Randomized controlled trial data indicates that addition of 1 hour of yoga, daily for 12 weeks to pharmacotherapy and CBT treatment protocol significantly improves anxiety scores (Cohen $d = 7.02$) [28]. Furthermore, addition of mindfulness-based cognitive therapy (MBCT) to pharmacotherapy treatment trial of patients with PD, was associated with greater improvement of both panic and anxiety symptoms [16].

Herbs, Botanicals, Supplements (HBS)

Clinicians may consider the addition of HBS as adjuncts to standard care taking into consideration factors such as safety, tolerability, cost, and patient preference.

Inositol

Data from a small, double-bling placebo-controlled crossover trial indicates that inositol**,** dosed at 12 grams was associated with significantly greater reduction in frequency of **PA**s. Specifically average number of weekly PAs was 10.1 (*SD* = 10) for placebo group and 2.4 (*SD* = 1) for group receiving inositol [7].

Nutritional Deficiencies

Deficiencies of vitamin B6 and iron may be associated with **PA** symptoms, as both are necessary to produce tryptophan, a precursor to serotonin [19]. Iron deficiency can commonly present without anemia in which case labs will demonstrate a low ferritin (< ~30 mg/dl or <100 mg/dl in states of chronic inflammation) and a low transferrin saturation (<20%) [2]. For patients presenting with risk factors for dietary deficiencies, B6 and iron levels can be checked. If deficiencies are identified, supplementation can be offered given potential benefits and low risk of harm.

Lastly, physicians should be aware that several medicinal herbs (Kava, Lavender, Ginkgo Biloba, and Ashwagandha) may be taken by the patients presenting with PD to alleviate symptoms. While limited data supports their use for anxiety disorders, there is a paucity of data focusing on **PD**.

Clinical Pearls

- Several brief screeners (see Table 3.1) offer efficient pathway to assessing **PD** symptoms
- In **PD**, **PA**s are often not triggered by stress, thus term “anxiety attack” may be inherently confusing to the patient.

- **PA**s activate **FFF** response which is an evolutionary “built in” mechanism to avoid danger. Built to protect, it produces uncomfortable symptoms which are not however dangerous.
- Avoidance is the primary mechanism for maintaining **PD**. It can take subtle forms. Successful treatment of PD is grounded in targeting avoidance behaviors. Physicians should be cognizant of its role and be mindful to not reinforce it.
- Targeting catastrophic interpretations of symptoms and teaching skills for self-regulation, while ensuring that patient understands “red flag” cardiac symptoms can pave way to effective **PD** management

Frequently Asked Questions

Question 1: *If someone is with me, I am not having **PA**s. Why is this?*
Answer: Having another person with you likely became a “safety signal” for you. While short term, this can be helpful and decrease worry, long-term this is likely contributing to **PD**. Always needing another person with you will make it harder to take care of yourself and can lead to strain on your relationships.

Question 2: *Should I purchase and use [relaxation gadget X]?*
Answer: Since **PA**s are often not triggered by stress, relaxation gadgets may not necessarily help with your symptoms. However, the gadget can become a safety signal for you, which in the long run creates more worry and can make you rely on it.

Question 3: *What should I do to make the **PA**s stop*?
Answer: There is a lot we can do to help manage your **PA**s. The first point to remember is that active avoidance of **PA**s can lead to having more not fewer episodes. The harder you try to get rid of them, the more frequent they become.

Case Vignette—Conclusion
Mr. V is back in the office to see Dr. L, 4 weeks after the diagnosis of **PD**.

Mr. V: *I looked over the **PD** materials and watched the videos. I understand what’s going on but it’s still scary. The more I try to avoid thinking about [**PA**s] and going places, the worse they get.*

Dr. L: *Many people with **PD** may do things to avoid **PA**s. However, this has the opposite effect often leading to more **panic attacks**.*

[Physician explains “Unwanted Party Guest” metaphor from **Emotional Acceptance** section]

Mr. V: *What do you think might help?*

Dr. L: *There is a technique called **diaphragmatic breathing** that can be used to calm the body and as a result the mind as well. It is a way to breathe using the muscles of your abdomen instead of those in the chest. Is it okay if we try it together now?*

Mr. V: *Yes, I am willing to give it a try.*

Dr. L: [Physician reviews **Diaphragmatic Breathing** steps]

Mr: V: *Well, what should I do if I cannot lower my heart rate? I think that's why I feel like I am having a heart attack.*

Dr. L: ***Diaphragmatic breathing*** *helps by slowing down breathing. If you are breathing slowly, what will happen to the heart?*

Mr. V: *The heart will slow down, just how it felt when we practiced.*

Dr. L: *That's exactly right and if the heart slows down the mind can calm down to help get you out of that* ***FFF*** *response.* (Mr. V nods). *Before our next appointment give the* ***diaphragmatic breathing*** *a try. It is important to practice daily, so that when a PA happens, you are well practiced with this skill.*

Resources

Source	Description	Link
Braive—YouTube channel	Video outlines **fight/flight/freeze** response to promote understanding of **PA** etiology	https://www.youtube.com/watch?v=SJhcn7Q0-LU&t=5s
National Institute of Mental Health **Panic Disorder:** What You Need to Know	Brief educational resource outlining symptoms, causes, diagnostics, treatment.	https://www.nimh.nih.gov/health/publications/panic-disorder-when-fear-overwhelms (English) https://www.nimh.nih.gov/health/publications/espanol/trastorno-de-panico-cuando-el-miedo-agobia (Spanish)
Craske, M.G. & Barlow, D. (2007). Mastery of your anxiety and panic. Patient Workbook (4th Ed). Treatments That Work. Oxford Academic. New York.	Forms and worksheets for CBT protocol for **PD** treatment. Support a range of activities including symptom tracking, cognitive disputation etc.	https://academic.oup.com/book/1262/chapter/140209000
American Psychological Association. Society of Clinical Psychology. Panic Disorder. Cognitive Behavioral Therapy for Panic Disorder	Site provides information on cognitive behavioral: self-help books, apps, handouts/worksheets, clinical manuals for **PD** treatment	https://div12.org/treatment/cognitive-behavioral-therapy-for-panic-disorder/#treatment-manuals
Digital therapeutics		
FreeSpira	FDA-cleared at-home treatment that addresses the symptoms associated with **PD**, panic/anxiety attacks. It corrects dysfunctional breathing associated with CO_2 hypersensitivity by training patients to stabilize their breathing.	https://dtxalliance.org/products/freespira/

(continued)

Source	Description	Link
HelloBetterPanic	Digital therapeutic program aimed at reducing the severity of symptoms associated with **PD** and agoraphobia. This digital intervention was developed and evaluated by a team of scientists and psychotherapists and is based on CBT	https://dtxalliance.org/products/hellobetter-panic-and-agoraphobia/

Metaphors for Panic/Fight Flight Freeze

Fire Drill—English

Panic attack is like a fire drill at work/school. Even though there is no fire, you must get ready to respond and quickly get out of the building. Your body does the same when it senses danger even if there isn't anything dangerous going on.

Simulacro de Incendio—Fire Drill, Spanish

Un ataque de pánico es como un simulacro de incendio en el trabajo o en la escuela. Aunque no haya un incendio real, debería prepararse para responder y salir rápidamente del edificio. Su cuerpo hace lo mismo cuando percibe un peligro, incluso aunque en realidad no haya nada peligroso ocurriendo.

Car in Neutral—English

Imagine a car that is in neutral gear. If you press gas, there will be a lot of noise—the engine will rev up and get hot. There will be a lot of noise but no movement. **Panic attack** is somewhat similar—there are many symptoms that indicate that you should be "going" but in reality, you are in neutral, since there is no danger to get away from.

Auto en Neutro—Car in Neutral, Spanish

Imagine un auto que esté en neutro. Si pisa el acelerador, hará mucho ruido: el motor se acelera y se calienta. Habrá mucho ruido, pero el auto no se moverá. Un ataque de pánico es algo parecido: hay muchos síntomas que indican que debería "estar en marcha", pero en realidad está en neutro, ya que no hay ningún peligro del cual escapar.

References

1. AlHadi AN, AlAteeq DA, Al-Sharif E, Bawazeer HM, Alanazi H, AlShomrani AT, Shuqdar RM, AlOwaybil R. An Arabic translation, reliability, and validation of Patient Health Questionnaire in a Saudi sample. Ann General Psychiatry. 2017;16:32. https://doi.org/10.1186/s12991-017-0155-1.
2. Al-Naseem A, Sallam A, Choudhury S, Thachil J. Iron deficiency without anaemia: a diagnosis that matters. Clin Med (Lond). 2021;21(2):107–13. https://doi.org/10.7861/clinmed.2020-0582.
3. American Psychiatric Association. Diagnostic and statistical manual of mental disorders (5th ed., text revised). Arlington, VA: Author; 2022.
4. Australian National University. Panic Disorder Screener (PADIS). n.d. Retrieved from: https://nceph.anu.edu.au/research/tools-resources/panic-disorder-screener-padis.
5. Barrera TL, Wilson KP, Norton PJ. The experience of panic symptoms across racial groups in a student sample. J Anxiety Disord. 2010;24(8):873–8. https://doi.org/10.1016/j.janxdis.2010.06.010.
6. Batterham PJ, Mackinnon AJ, Christensen H. The panic disorder screener (PADIS): development of an accurate and brief population screening tool. Psychiatry Res. 2015;228(1):72–6. https://doi.org/10.1016/j.psychres.2015.04.016.
7. Benjamin J, Levine J, Fux M, Aviv A, Levy D, Belmaker RH. Double-blind, placebo-controlled, crossover trial of inositol treatment for panic disorder. Am J Psychiatry. 1995;152(7):1084–6. https://doi.org/10.1176/ajp.152.7.1084.
8. Bilet T, Olsen T, Andersen JR, Martinsen EW. Cognitive behavioral group therapy for panic disorder in a general clinical setting: a prospective cohort study with 12 to 31-years follow-up. BMC Psychiatry. 2020;20(1):259. Published 2020 May 24. https://doi.org/10.1186/s12888-020-02679-w.
9. Craske MG, Barlow D. Mastery of your anxiety and panic. Therapist Guide (4th Ed). Treatments that work. New York: Oxford University Press; 2007.
10. Fuste G, Gil MÁ, López-Solà C, Rosado S, Bonillo A, Pailhez G, Bulbena A, Pérez V, Fullana MA. Psychometric properties of the Spanish version of the panic disorder severity scale. Span J Psychol. 2018;21:E5. https://doi.org/10.1017/sjp.2018.6.
11. Gaudlitz K, Plag J, Dimeo F, Ströhle A. Aerobic exercise training facilitates the effectiveness of cognitive behavioral therapy in panic disorder. Depress Anxiety. 2015;32(3):221–8. https://doi.org/10.1002/da.22337.
12. Harvard Medical School, 2007. National Comorbidity Survey (NCS). 2017. Retrieved from https://www.hcp.med.harvard.edu/ncs/index.php. Data Table 1: Lifetime prevalence DSM-IV/WMH-CIDI disorders by sex and cohort.
13. Hayes SC, Smith S. Get Out of Your Mind and Into Your Life: The New Acceptance & Commitment Therapy. Oakland, CA: New Harbinger Publications; 2005.
14. Jayakody K, Gunadasa S, Hosker C. Exercise for anxiety disorders: systematic review. Br J Sports Med. 2014;48(3):187–96. https://doi.org/10.1136/bjsports-2012-091287.
15. Kessler RC, Chiu WT, Jin R, Ruscio AM, Shear K, Walters EE. The epidemiology of panic attacks, panic disorder, and agoraphobia in the National Comorbidity Survey Replication. Arch Gen Psychiatry. 2006;63(4):415–424. https://doi.org/10.1001/archpsyc.63.4.415.
16. Kim B, Lee SH, Kim YW, Choi TK, Yook K, Suh SY, Cho SJ, Yook KH. Effectiveness of a mindfulness-based cognitive therapy program as an adjunct to pharmacotherapy in patients with panic disorder. J Anxiety Disord. 2010;24(6):590–5. https://doi-org.ezproxy.cul.columbia.edu/10.1016/j.janxdis.2010.03.019.
17. Lippman D, Stump M, Veazey E, Guimarães ST, Rosenfeld R, Kelly JH, Ornish D, Katz DL. Foundations of lifestyle medicine and its evolution. Mayo Clin Proc Innov Qual Outcomes. 2024;8(1):97–111. https://doi.org/10.1016/j.mayocpiqo.2023.11.004.
18. Liu X, Xu T, Chen D, Yang C, Wang P, Huang X, Cheng W, Shen Y, Liu Q, Wang Z. Reliability, validity and cut-off score of the Chinese version of the panic disorder severity scale self-

report form in patients with panic disorder. BMC Psychiatry. 2020;20(1):170. https://doi.org/10.1186/s12888-020-02560-w.
19. Mikawa Y, Mizobuchi S, Egi M, Morita K. Low serum concentrations of vitamin B6 and iron are related to panic attack and hyperventilation attack. Acta Med Okayama. 2013;67(2):99–104. https://doi.org/10.18926/AMO/49668.
20. Muñoz-Navarro R, Cano-Vindel A, Wood CM, Ruíz-Rodríguez P, Medrano LA, Limonero JT, Tomás-Tomás P, Gracia-Gracia I, Dongil-Collado E, Iruarrizaga MI, PsicAP Research Group. The PHQ-PD as a screening tool for panic disorder in the primary care setting in Spain. PLoS One. 2016;11(8):e0161145. https://doi.org/10.1371/journal.pone.0161145.
21. Novopsych. Panic Disorder Severity Scale. n.d. Retrieved June 5, 2025 from https://novopsych.com.au/assessments/anxiety/panic-disorder-severity-scale-pdss/.
22. Pfizer. Welcome to the Patient Health Questionnaire (PHQ) Screeners: screener overview. n.d. Retrieved June 5, 2025 from https://www.phqscreeners.com/select-screener.
23. Pompoli A, Furukawa TA, Efthimiou O, Imai H, Tajika A, Salanti G. Dismantling cognitive-behaviour therapy for panic disorder: a systematic review and component network meta-analysis. Psychol Med. 2018;48(12):1945–1953. https://doi.org/10.1017/S0033291717003919.
24. Saeed SA, Cunningham K, Bloch RM. Depression and anxiety disorders: benefits of exercise, yoga, and meditation. Am Fam Physician. 2019;99(10):620–7.
25. Shear MK, Brown TA, Barlow DH, Money R, Sholomskas DE, Woods SW, Gorman JM, Papp LA. Multicenter collaborative panic disorder severity scale. Am J Psychiatry. 1997;154(11):1571–5. https://doi.org/10.1176/ajp.154.11.1571.
26. Spitzer RL, Kroenke K, Williams JB. Validation and utility of a self-report version of PRIME-MD: the PHQ primary care study. Primary care evaluation of mental disorders. Patient Health Questionnaire. JAMA. 1999;282(18):1737–44. https://doi.org/10.1001/jama.282.18.1737.
27. Wuyek LA, Antony MM, McCabe RE. Psychometric properties of the panic disorder severity scale: clinician-administered and self-report versions. Clin Psychol Psychother. 2011;18(3):234–43. https://doi.org/10.1002/cpp.703.
28. Yadla VS, Patil NJ, Kamarthy P, Matti MR. Effect of integrated yoga as an adjuvant to standard care for panic disorder: a randomized control trial study. Cureus. 2024;16(1):e53286. https://doi.org/10.7759/cureus.53286.
29. Zhang D, Lee EKP, Mak ECW, Ho CY, Wong SYS. Mindfulness-based interventions: an overall review. Br Med Bull. 2021;138(1):41–57. https://doi.org/10.1093/bmb/ldab005.

Chapter 4
Posttraumatic Stress Disorder (PTSD)

Nataliya Pilipenko, Krishna M. Desai, and Aury Garcia

Case Vignette

Ms. B is a 29-year-old woman with a history of cluster headaches, type 1 diabetes, and a gunshot wound to the right leg in the setting of intimate partner violence.

Ms. B: *Three years ago, my partner and I got into another argument. Things got out of hand. He threatened to kill me, got his gun out. He threatened me before, but never like this. I started running and then my leg just gave out. I fell! (closes her eyes, begins to sob). I thought he was going to shoot me in the head (continues sobbing). I am reliving what happened that day, every single day since. Noises, sounds—all scare me. I can hardly watch the news—too many shootings! I can't sleep because of the nightmares. I try to put that day behind me, but I can't.*

Dr. C: *That was terrifying! It sounds like you are reliving that day. Time is passing but you are not feeling better.*

Ms. B: *Yes, you are right. I stopped hanging out with family and friends. Just go to work and come straight home. Always on edge. I lash out at people over the smallest things.*

N. Pilipenko (✉)
Center for Family and Community Medicine, Department of Medicine, Columbia University Irving Medical Center/New York Presbyterian Hospital, New York, NY, USA

Department of Psychiatry, Columbia University Irving Medical Center, New York, NY, USA
e-mail: np2615@cumc.columbia.edu

K. M. Desai
Center for Family and Community Medicine, Department of Medicine, Columbia University Irving Medical Center/New York Presbyterian Hospital, New York, NY, USA

Center for Neuroinflammatory and Somatic Disorders, Department of Psychiatry, Columbia University Irving Medical Center/New York Presbyterian Hospital, New York, NY, USA

A. Garcia
Center for Family and Community Medicine, Department of Medicine, Columbia University Irving Medical Center/New York Presbyterian Hospital, New York, NY, USA

N. Pilipenko, K. M. Desai (eds.), *8 Conditions Primary Care Clinicians Dread to Treat*, https://doi.org/10.1007/978-3-032-12819-5_4

Dr. C: *Has anything helped with these symptoms?*
Ms. B: *No. I try so hard to put this behind me, but I can't. I am not sure what to do to snap out of it. That's why I am here today.*
Dr. C: *I would like to propose that we spend today's visit to assess your symptoms, talk about the diagnosis as well as ways to help you move forward. What do you think about this?*
Ms. B: *I suppose that's the only option. I tried to avoid this topic for a long time.*
Dr. C: [Discussed Message #1]*.

Note. In this case, DSM-5-TR criterion for traumatic events is clearly met (threatened death, actual serious injury). In cases when specifics of a traumatic event are clear, assessment should precede delivery of Message #1).

Diagnosis: Brief Description

Diagnostic criteria for PTSD require direct experiencing, witnessing, or exposure to a traumatic event, defined as "actual or threatened death, serious injury or sexual violence" [2, p. 301]. Exposure can take place via work activities (e.g., police work) or by learning of a **trauma** occurring to a "close family member or a friend".

Subsequently to the **trauma**, at least one intrusive symptom (e.g., distressing memories, dreams, dissociative reactions, flashbacks) and at least one **avoidance** symptom (efforts to avoid **trauma**-related memories, thoughts and feelings, reminders) must be present. Additionally, at least two symptoms from each of the following groups must also be present/develop subsequently to the **trauma:**

- Negative alterations in cognitions or mood: amnesia of important aspects of **trauma**, negative beliefs about oneself, others, or the world; distorted, blame-related cognitions about causes or consequences of **trauma**; persistent negative emotional state; decreased interest in activity engagement; feelings of detachment or estrangement from others, inability to experience positive affect.
- Changes in arousal and reactivity: anger or irritability; recklessness or self-destructive behaviors; hypervigilance; exaggerated startle response; concentration difficulties; or sleep difficulties.

Symptom duration must exceed 1 month, be associated with distress and/or impairment. Please refer to DSM-5-TR [2] for information pertaining to the differential diagnostic considerations.

Prevalence, Risk Factors, and Disparities

According to the DSM-5-TR [2], the lifetime prevalence of PTSD among U.S. adults is 6.8%. However, caution must be exercised to avoid conflation of **PTSD** with exposure to traumatic events, since epidemiological data shows that 70% of the general population experience lifetime **trauma** event, as defined by DSM-5-TR criteria [4]. Nevertheless, physicians should be mindful that certain patients may be at an elevated risk of **trauma** exposure due to their profession (e.g. military, law enforcement) or other characteristics (e.g. pregnancy status, age, place of residence). Nonetheless, while several research studies link the number of traumatic events to increased **PTSD** risk, others contend that **trauma**-related cognitions (rather than number of events) are primary drivers behind morbidity [19, 22].

In primary care (PC), **PTSD** estimates range between 2–39% [12].

In the U.S., the lowest adjusted estimated prevalence rates of **PTSD** are reported by Asians, and the highest by African Americans, with Afro-Caribbeans, White, and Latino groups endorsing similar prevalence rates [1].

Symptom Assessment Tools

Table 4.1 presents three widely used **PTSD** screeners. Specifically, Primary Care-**PTSD**-5 (PC-**PTSD**-5, [32]) is a PC-validated screener. The **PTSD** Checklist (PCL-5, [5]) is a longer tool, which allows for more in-depth symptom assessment and nuanced tracking. Finally, the Clinician Administered **PTSD** Scale for Children and Adolescents (CAPS-CA-5, [35]) can be used for children ages 7 or older. Please see **Assess and Monitor Symptoms** section for further discussion.

Table 4.1 PTSD Screening Tools

Screener name	Items #	Rating scale scoring	Cut offs	Assessment timeline	Availability	Psychometric properties	Non-English Versions?
Primary care PTSD 5 (PC-PTSD-5)	5	Binary [32] 0 = No 1 = Yes	Cut off point of 4 balances false negatives and positives, cut off point of 3 is recommended for women [32]	1 month [32]	Open access [32]	Diagnostic accuracy [32] AUC = .94; 95% confidence interval (CI): .91–.97 Cut score of 3 maximized sensitivity (κ [1]) [32] = .93; standard error (SE) = .04; 95% CI: .85–1.00 Cut score of 4 maximized efficiency (κ[0.5] [32] = .63; SE = .05; 95% CI: .53–0.73 Cut score of 5 maximized specificity (κ[0]) [32] = .70; SE = .08; 95% CI: .55–.85	Chinese [16]

PTSD checklist 5 (PCL-5)[a]	20 [5]	5-point Likert [11] 0 = not at all to 4 = extremely	Score of 31–33 [11] out of 80 is indicative of probable PTSD	1 week [11] or 1 month	Open access [11]	Initial based on trauma exposed college students [5] Internal consistency (α = .94) Test-retest reliability (r = .82) Convergent (rs = .74–.85) Discriminant validity (rs = .31–.60)	Arabic [17], Chinese [27], Spanish [6], Tagalog [13]
[a]3 versions of PCL-5 are available—military, civilian or specific trauma							
Clinician Administered PTSD Scale for Children and Adolescents-5 (CAPS-CA-5)	30 [33]	5-point Likert [33] Symptoms are rated as absent or present, then further rated on intensity and frequency, and combined into a severity score from: 0 = Absent 4 = Extreme/ incapacitating for each item	PTSD diagnosis is determined by dichotomizing symptoms as present or absent then following DSM-5 diagnostic criteria. Present if score is 2 = moderate or higher[a]	1 month [33]	Copyrighted [33]	Good internal consistency (α = .52–.82 in children ages 7–14) [35] (α = .72–.9 in children older than 14) [14]	Arabic (Tunesian dialect) [21]

[a]Please refer to citation 10 below for more details on scoring and cut-offs

Non-pharmacological Conceptualization: What to Say to the Patient?

Message #1: Symptoms Are Understandable and Appropriate Responses to Trauma

PTSD symptoms are appropriate reactions to extreme negative emotions experienced during traumatic event(s). When a traumatic event occurs, a person's primary goal is to successfully survive it, and there is no time or opportunity to process these events as they happen. Later, however, **trauma**-associated emotions (specifically: fear, guilt, shame and anger) are activated in association with **trauma** memories and reminders (e.g., smells, physical sensations, reminiscent circumstances) and lead to **re-experiencing**. **Re-experiencing** results in distress and may lead individuals to feel and behave as though the traumatic event is happening again. Understandably, this results in efforts to avoid both **trauma** memories and associated reminders. **Avoidance** of **trauma** can take many forms: staying away from others, using substances to numb emotions, limiting activities. However, in the long run, **avoidance** results in stronger feelings of distress as well as problems with relationships, work performance, and others.

It is important to remember, that unlike the actual **trauma**, memories (albeit upsetting) are not dangerous, but ongoing **avoidance** contributes to feelings of unsafety. Concurrently, two other groups of problems emerge: negative changes in thoughts, feelings and relationships (e.g., blaming self or others, low mood, hopelessness) and hyperarousal (e.g., feeling on edge, poor sleep, being irritable). Both worsen symptoms and further interfere with daily living.

Why? Trauma is associated with fear, guilt, shame and anger [42] which create a barrier to discussing both the events and their impact. Additionally, patients suffering from **PTSD** may worry that their symptoms are highly unusual because they are experiencing extreme distress in absence of a current threat. This worry may be particularly salient for patients who experience delay in onset of **PTSD** symptoms (6 months or longer). Furthermore, patients are likely to be exposed to (and possibly endorse) explanations of **trauma** and post-**trauma** reactions which directly or indirectly blame themselves for the event(s) (See **Address Just World Explanations** section for further discussion). Synergistically, these factors build significant barriers for care of patients suffering from **PTSD**. Thus, it is important to communicate about **PTSD** symptoms and connections between symptom groups (e.g., **re-experiencing** and **avoidance**) clearly and openly. This discussion does not require patients to discuss their **trauma**; however, it does communicate understanding of illness experience thus supporting trust.

Message #2: Address "Just World" and "Silver Lining" Explanations Directly

We live in a dangerous and unpredictable world, where terrible things happen daily. This is frightening for all of us. To make the world feel safer, people often rely on "**Just World**" explanations stating that somehow the **trauma** was a consequence of the victim's own character, action, or inaction. Additionally, to make sense of negative events, many people rely on the "**Silver lining**" explanations—that all bad events have a positive aspect. Both "**Just World**" and "**Silver lining**" explanations have a fundamental problem: they fail to assign the responsibility for the **trauma** appropriately. While the former blames the victim, the latter obfuscates responsibility for the harm done. Both explanations fail to openly acknowledge that it is the perpetrator who is responsible for the **trauma**, not the victim.

Why? Societal handling of **trauma** rests on the "dynamic balance between containment and expression" whereby victims are encouraged "to say just so much about what happened, but not too much" [18, p. 2]. However, Littleton [26] notes that negative reactions to **trauma** disclosure (i.e., attempts to distract victims from **trauma**, victim-blaming) predicted maladaptive coping, self-blame, and negative self-cognitions. Thus, addressing reactions to **trauma** is an important component of **trauma** care.

While "**Just World**" belief serves an important adaptive function as it allows individuals "to confront [their] physical and social environment as though they were stable and orderly" [23, p. 1030]. According to this belief: "Victims can deserve their fate as a consequence of having a "bad" character or as a consequence of engaging in "bad" acts" (p. 1031). For in-depth overview and research examining this belief, see Lerner and Miller [23]. While "**Just World**" belief benefits social stability, it serves to protect the perpetrator rather than support the victim.

While **trauma** can potentially result in posttraumatic growth, including perceptions of new possibilities, positive relationship changes, enhanced perceptions of personal strength, spiritual change, and appreciation of life [37], the "**Silver lining**" rationalizations should be approached with great caution to avoid shifting focus away from victim's needs, harm done, and perpetrator's responsibility.

Message #3: Address Relational Aspects of Trauma and Avoidance

Trauma experiences always involve other people. While at the time of the **trauma** event, the victim may be alone, responses include relationships with others (present or absent). Thus, within **trauma** experience, there is a perpetrator (person(s) responsible for harm) as well as by-standers (those who could either not stop the perpetrator or chose not to do so). After a traumatic event, the human mind aims to make sense of the event(s) and navigate new situations. Frequently, **trauma**-related thoughts (e.g., **re-experiencing**) and behaviors (e.g., **avoidance**) emerge in response to **trauma** reminders to promote safety and control negative emotions.

It is important for both the physician and the patient to be aware and mindful about effect of past **trauma** sequelae in shaping current reactions and relationships. For example, a patient who has sexual **trauma**, may feel anxious or angry with a physician when a gynecological exam is mentioned– or may skip the visit altogether. Alternatively, **trauma** may have resulted as help was too slow to arrive. Consequently, patients may feel very anxious or angry when even minor delays (e.g., unanswered phone calls, delays in discussing test results) arise. Without an understanding of the patient's **trauma** history, these reactions can appear out of proportion to the event and leave care teams confused and frustrated.

The following statement can be helpful in proactively addressing such challenges: "During our work together, things will happen that will bring up your **trauma** memories. Maybe I (or a member of your care team) will say or do something that will bring up feelings and thoughts about **trauma**, or a situation may also occur that will remind you of it. If this happens, please let me know. While it is never my intention to upset you, given that you are the only person who will ever fully know what happened, it might not be possible for me or my team to fully anticipate **trauma** reminders. Please let me know if you are finding yourself being reminded of **trauma** or trying to avoid something so that we can discuss how to best navigate the situation to move forward."

Why? Relationship and relatedness challenges are central to post **trauma** sequelae. **Trauma** survivors may believe that because of traumatic event(s) they are different from others, their experiences cannot be understood, or that they will be rejected [8]. Understanding broad principles of **trauma**'s operation in the context of medical care is critical to physician's ability to treat patients with **PTSD**. Please note that this discussion requires no knowledge of the **trauma** specifics, nor does it require for such details to be elicited.

Johnson and Lubin [18] note the following four axioms of **trauma** treatment. First, trauma schemas (patterns of emotions and cognitions) are always relational, and thus are activated in context of **trauma** victim's relationships with others (including medical care team). Second, the story of the traumatic event(s) is always incomplete. Thus, physicians should assume that they do not know the full story and thus cannot fully anticipate a patient's reactions. Third, **avoidance** of **trauma** will be ongoing and both patient and the physician will be participating in it. **Avoidance** should be assumed as always operating. Finally, **trauma** schemata are activated when a patient is reminded of the **trauma** to decrease **trauma**-related negative emotions. This process will likely bring about behaviors which may be misperceived as irrational, angry, or otherwise dysfunctional. Understanding current reactions through axioms of **trauma** treatment can prepare both patient and physician for effective partnership.

Given the complexity of **trauma** for both patients and physicians (and care teams), it may be tempting to dismiss **trauma** as a factor peripheral to medical care.

However, **PTSD** is associated with multiple outcomes which are highly relevant to physical health. Specifically: increased medical illness burden, greater healthcare utilization, poor quality of life, and functional impairment [12, 31]. Furthermore, **PTSD** diagnosis and sub-diagnostic **PTSD** symptoms are associated with a greater number of medical conditions, particularly pain, GI, and cardiac symptoms [31]. Reassuringly, however, when **PTSD** is treated, better medical illness management and symptom control can be achieved [40].

Case Vignette—Continued

Ms. B returns to see Dr. C in 4 weeks. Her PC-PTSD-5 score (administered at the end of the first visit) was 4. PCL-5 was administered. Total score was 47, indicative of probable **PTSD** [38]. The patient was also provided with educational material (See Resources) which describe symptoms of **PTSD**. Dr. C asked Ms. B to review these educational materials before this visit.

Ms. B: (looking visibly frustrated) *You know, I almost did not come to see you today. The front desk staff really got on my nerves. I sat there for ages, and they just would not budge to give me my paperwork! I won't be treated this way!*

Dr. C: *I apologize about this delay at the front desk. I hear that this did upset you a lot! I will bring this up at our staff meeting to see why there was a delay and what we can do to prevent this going forward. I do apologize though.*

Ms. B: *Ok. Thank you.*

Dr. C: *Since we talked about your trauma history during our last appointment, I just want to ask if what happened at the front desk, may have somehow reminded you about being shot?*

Ms. B: *I never really thought about it. Your staff really do need to get on with what they are doing.*

Dr. C: Absolutely. I just want to check in to make sure that we are not missing anything trauma related. Sometimes it can happen.

Mr. B: *Well… (pauses). After I was shot, I called 911. They kept asking stupid questions and did not seem to understand or care that he almost killed me. They did not care how scared I was. I was terrified that he was going to come back and shoot me. This time, in the head! I was crying and they were telling me to "stay calm." Maybe waiting here last time and seeing how your staff are in no hurry triggered me? When I walked up to them, they were like "stay calm, it's not a big deal."*

Dr. C: *It sounds like the delay may have been a trigger. I am glad you were able to return to see me.* [Physician outlines Message #3]

Ms. B: *I understand. Once you talk about my reactions in this way, I do not feel like I am crazy. Like what I have been through explains my reactions even though I am overreacting.*

Non-pharmacological Treatment Options: What Can Be Done?

Unlike other conditions covered in this book, there is a limited armamentarium which is available to physicians for **PTSD** interventions, as current treatment protocols are built on expectation of ongoing, regular engagement and participation in treatment sessions of significant duration. However, utilization of Messages 1–3 (previously outlined) is central and can be conceptualized as therapeutic as these help to recognize and address intra- and interpersonal components of **PTSD**. Several techniques may be further helpful in caring for patients with **PTSD**.

1. **Assess and Monitor Symptoms**

   Research suggests that **PTSD** is poorly detected and documented within PC settings [9, 25]. While reasons behind these practices are multifaceted, its outcome is likely contributing to ongoing challenges with **PTSD** treatment, as unidentified conditions cannot receive clinical attention and management.

   Given the impact of **PTSD** symptoms upon physical, psychological and interpersonal functioning, monitoring its symptoms is an important task, regardless of whether the patient is receiving treatment (pharmacotherapy or psychotherapy) or not. In case when either treatment is received, symptom tracking is an important measurement of treatment success. While if the patient is not in treatment for **PTSD**, screening scores (especially if elevated) can be discussed as moderators of overall health status and quality of life thus fostering goals of care discussion.

   Currently the United States Preventative Task force does not issue standardized recommendations for initial and follow-up screening for **PTSD**. While 6-item PC-PTSD-5 ([32], see Table 4.1) offers an efficient initial screening option, physicians should be mindful that tools with a small number of items (that ideal for initial screening), may be ineffective tools for tracking treatment progress. This is due to the small range of scores (in case of PC-PTSD-5 range 0–5) restricting ability to note symptom changes over time. However, screening tools with more items (such as **Posttraumatic stress disorder** Checklist for DSM-5, PCL-5, [41]) will offer more robust longitudinal assessment of symptom changes.

   Given the prevalence of trauma events and their impact, using PC-**PTSD**-5 at least once with all patients can pave way to more trauma-focused care. If significant symptoms emerge, use Message #1 to discuss symptoms and diagnostic impressions. If the diagnosis of **PTSD** is established, initial PCL screening administration can be considered to establish a baseline. Thereafter, PCL can be used to determine if the symptoms and their impact are changing.
2. **Continuously Normalize and Educate About Symptoms and Their Impact**

   Messages 1–3 outlined earlier in this chapter offer foundation to both diagnostic discussion and interpersonal management of **PTSD** sequelae. However, it is important that discussions about **PTSD** are normalized and continue throughout the treatment. Communication of findings based on screening tools, inquiry about domains of functioning which are affected by **PTSD**, and open discussion about **PTSD** treatment and its consequences.

For example, a physician might ask about progress of **PTSD** therapy as well as any connections which a patient observes between overall health management and trauma treatment. Such questions can communicate acknowledgement of **PTSD** symptoms as ongoing factors in a patient's life and healthcare decisions, reduce negative emotions (via ongoing exposure) and target trauma-related negative cognitions (e.g. isolation, rejection).

Psychotherapy for PTSD

APA's Clinical Practice Guidelines for treatment of **PTSD** (2017, 2025), note the following three EBPs for **PTSD**: CBT [29], Cognitive Processing Therapy (CPT, Resick et al. [34]) and Prolonged Exposure (PE, Foa et al. [10]). A systematic review and meta-analysis of CBT for **PTSD** notes the within-group effect sizes (ES) for **PTSD**-severity at post-treatment (1.75), and follow-up (1.70), on average six months post-treatment, were large [30]. Meta-analytic findings indicate that CPT "outperformed inactive control conditions on **PTSD** outcome measures at posttreatment (mean *Hedges' g* = 1.24) and follow-up (mean *Hedges' g* = 0.90)" and demonstrated lasting benefits across a range of outcomes, although effect sizes of reported trials vary [3]. Finally, Bradley and colleagues [7] report that 53% of patients who initiate PE no longer meet diagnostic criteria for the **PTSD**, and the rate of diagnostic change increases to 68% among individuals who complete treatment.

Integrative Medicine Interventions and Techniques

Is it important for physicians to be aware of Integrative Medicine (IM) strategies for trauma as a significant number of patients diagnosed with **PTSD** utilize these approaches [24].

Mind-Body Practices (MBP): Mindfulness-Based Stress Reduction

Overall, MBPs may be helpful for trauma-related **avoidance**, negative cognitions, and in regulating physiological symptoms associated with these responses [20]. Meta analysis findings demonstrated that eight week-long mindfulness-based stress reduction (MBSR) treatments reduce the **PTSD** symptoms with a moderately positive effect *(g = .46, 95% CI [0.31, 0.62])* [28].

Movement-Based Interventions (MBI): Yoga

Movement-based interventions (**yoga**, tai-chi, and qigong) involve connecting movement, breathing, relaxation, and non-judgmental awareness of the present moment experience. A systematic review and meta-analysis demonstrated that yoga-based interventions *(g = 0.91, 95% CI* [0.38, 1.45]) were associated with significant and greater symptom improvement, as compared to exercise *g = 13, 95% CI* [−.09, .34]) [39].

Additionally, MBIs may benefit patients overall via promoting engagement in physical activity, patient empowerment through self-care tools, and social connectedness. These techniques carry low risk of harm and can be offered as part of a multi-faceted patient-centered treatment approach. Free online tools and low-cost community programs may be particularly valuable.

Acupuncture

Acupuncture holds promise in advancing **PTSD** treatment as it regulates the structure and components of several brain areas, neuroendocrine system, and signaling pathways [36] and is well tolerated [15].

Meta analytic findings by Tang et al. [36] indicate that **acupuncture** is not only associated with decreased **PTSD** symptom scores but can also outperform both pharmacotherapy and psychotherapy across several symptom measures. Furthermore, randomized control trial data suggests that verum application (proper needling technique) is associated with large effect size in **PTSD** symptom improvement (*Cohen's d* = 1.17) while sham treatment is associated with only moderate effect size (*Cohen's d* = 0.67) [15].

Physicians can use the following script to recommend **acupuncture**: *"**Acupuncture** uses very thin, hair-like needles which are placed on specific points of the body. Research shows that it can regulate parts of the brain involved in stress and emotion. Most people tolerate the treatment very well with few side effects. They describe the sensation of the needles as light pressure, tingling, or warmth, and many people feel deeply relaxed during treatment. For people with post-traumatic stress disorder (**PTSD**), **acupuncture** can reduce hyperarousal, improve sleep, ease irritability, and improve overall mood. **Acupuncture** can be safely used alongside therapy and medications. At first, it is done once or twice a week, and many people start to notice improvements after several sessions."*

Physicians can help patients find a licensed acupuncturist by using national registries such as National Certification Commission for **Acupuncture** and Oriental Medicine (NCCAOM) and American Society of Acupuncturists (ASA).

Clinical Pearls

- Brief screeners for **PTSD** (e.g., PC-**PTSD**-5) offer efficient and effective identification of patients with **PTSD** symptoms. Longer screeners (e.g., PCL) should be used for symptom tracking over time.
- Discuss symptoms of **PTSD** as understandable reactions to traumatic events which include **re-experiencing** and **avoidance** of trauma-related reminders.
- Discuss and manage interpersonal aspects of trauma-related beliefs ("**Just World**", "**Silver Lining**").
- Expect that **PTSD** symptoms will impact interpersonal relationships and approach these as expected part of trauma care.
- Mindfulness-based stress reduction, **yoga** and **acupuncture** can be recommended for amelioration of **PTSD** symptoms.

Frequently Asked Questions

Question 1: *I do not want to see anyone [any other physician/provider] but you I do not want to talk about what happened and explain my [trauma] again.*

Answer: Talking about trauma is upsetting. Living through a trauma makes it difficult to trust others so many patients do not feel at ease at the thought of meeting new providers. We need to remember a few things though. First, unless you are talking to your therapist, you do not need to recount details of what has happened to you. Secondly, meeting new members of the care team and building relationships with them, can be beneficial as this will allow you to know that despite the trauma that happened, there are many people who will treat you well and will not let you down.

Question 2: *I have learned to accept [trauma], but I feel very angry and upset all the time. What can I do about that?*

Answer: If your anger emerged after or got significantly worse after your [trauma], it may be connected to **PTSD**. Especially since we know that anger, irritability, being impulsive, and trouble connecting with others are **PTSD** symptoms. My recommendation is to discuss your **PTSD** diagnosis and your treatment preferences with your therapist. You may decide that addressing your trauma is not something that you want to do now (or ever) and you just want to focus on behaviorally controlling your anger. However, if your anger is the result of **PTSD**, learning techniques for anger management without addressing the trauma itself is going to be a 'band aid' solution which may not work consistently.

Question 3: *My husband was diagnosed with **PTSD**, and I do not know how to help him. What should I do?*

Answer: Living with someone who has **PTSD** can be challenging and there is no simple recipe or solution. However, there are specialized resources which can offer more support. Would you like me to provide you with this information?

[offer National Centers for **PTSD** resources for Family and Friends, see Resources].

Case Vignette—Conclusion

Ms. B returns for follow-up with Dr. C. It has been 6 weeks since the initial visit. Although Ms. B reviewed educational materials and was provided with psychotherapy referral, she has not pursued it stating that she needs "more time to think it over." Ms. B's PCL-5 score at the time of the appointment is 50.

Ms. B: I have been *down since our last meeting. My mom made a comment about me getting shot because I provoked [partner] at the time. She always tells me what a great guy he is and how I must have given him a reason. I tried to speak to my cousin about it, but she just said it was part of God's plan. I just feel like I deserve it.*

Dr. C: [Discussed Message #2].

Ms. B: *What exactly are our next steps? I can't keep living like this.*

Dr. C: In general, you have three options. The first one is to wait to see if your symptoms lessen without an intervention. But you have been waiting for three years now, and they are not improving, correct?

Ms. B: (nods).

Dr. C: *This leaves us with three options: medications, psychotherapy or a combination of both. I know that you have been thinking about therapy but have not yet moved forward with setting it up. We can also discuss medications which can help to manage **PTSD** symptoms. The choice is yours.*

Ms. B: *I am just too scared that if I am going to start talking about it, I will come completely undone.*

Dr. C: *This is a common concern. Memories, flashbacks are very upsetting, and it feels like therapy will just be too overwhelming.*

Ms. B: *Yes. I don't know how people can stand it.*

Dr. C: *There are several important aspects of therapy that can help people tolerate talking about trauma. Do you want me to describe these?*

Ms. B: *Ok. Tell me.*

Dr. C: *First, you and your therapist will agree on the specific therapy approach, and you will have a chance to understand how and why it will work. Unlike your traumatic experience, you will be in control. Although you tried to forget and move on, your memories are still there, even though you are doing your best to avoid them. Unfortunately, **avoidance** does not make the memories go away and therapy targets this process in a way that works for many people.*

Ms. B: *I hear you. I will plan to call a few therapists tomorrow and schedule a first visit.*

Dr. C: Is there anything that I can do to support you?

Ms. B: *Will you be able to speak to my therapist, once I find one?*

Dr. C: *Absolutely! Once you decide on a specific therapist, you will just need to sign a form giving us permission to speak with each other. You can sign this form in my office or with your therapist.*

Ms. B: Ok. It will make me feel a little better.

Dr. C: *Sounds like a plan. If you want to re-visit medications for* ***PTSD*** *symptoms management—just let me know. If it's ok with you, I would like for us to keep monitoring your* ***PTSD*** *symptoms when you come back to see me. What do you think about this plan?*

Ms. B: *That's ok. Let's keep tracking them to see how things are going.*

Resources

Source	Description	Link
National Centers for PTSD	Website offers a range of resources to support patients, families and providers	Treatment decision aid: https://www.PTSD.va.gov/appvid/decisionaid_public.asp Screening tools: https://www.PTSD.va.gov/professional/assessment/screens/index.asp Resources for the families: https://www.PTSD.va.gov/family/how_help.asp Educational videos about various psychotherapies: https://www.PTSD.va.gov/appvid/video/index.asp Resources in Spanish https://www.PTSD.va.gov/spanish/index.asp
Substance Abuse and Mental Health Services Administration	Tips for survivors of disaster and other traumatic event (Spanish)	https://library.samhsa.gov/sites/default/files/PEP20-01-01-025.pdf
American Psychological Association	Clinical practice guideline for the treatment of PTSD in adults Resource includes: Treatment manuals Training opportunities	https://www.apa.org/PTSD-guideline/resources
American Psychological Association, Society of Clinical Psychology	Offers review (including evaluation of the strength of supporting evidence) for various PTSD-focused psychotherapies Click on each treatment to learn more. When available, information about treatment manuals and bibliotherapy is provided	https://div12.org/treatments/?_sfm_related_diagnosis=8142
Yoga with Adriene	**Yoga** For Post Traumatic Stress. 45 min	https://www.youtube.com/watch?v=TqVSwY8y3UY
Digital Therapeutics		
FreeSpira	Evidence summary: https://beonbrand.getbynder.com/m/98cca0245f0d647b/original/Digital-Therapeutic-Products-for-Post-traumatic-Stress-Disorder-and-Panic-Disorder.pdf	https://dtxalliance.org/products/freespira/

References

1. Alegría M, Fortuna LR, Lin JY, Norris FH, Gao S, Takeuchi DT, Jackson JS, Shrout PE, Valentine A. Prevalence, risk, and correlates of posttraumatic stress disorder across ethnic and racial minority groups in the United States. Med Care. 2013;51(12):1114–23. https://doi.org/10.1097/MLR.0000000000000007.
2. American Psychiatric Association. Diagnostic and statistical manual of mental disorders. 5th ed., text revised ed. Arlington: Author; 2022.
3. Asmundson GJG, Thorisdottir AS, Roden-Foreman JW, et al. A meta-analytic review of cognitive processing therapy for adults with posttraumatic stress disorder. Cogn Behav Ther. 2019;48(1):1–14. https://doi.org/10.1080/16506073.2018.1522371.
4. Benjet C, Bromet E, Karam EG, Kessler RC, McLaughlin KA, Ruscio AM, Shahly V, Stein DJ, Petukhova M, Hill E, Alonso J, Atwoli L, Bunting B, Bruffaerts R, Caldas-de-Almeida JM, de Girolamo G, Florescu S, Gureje O, Huang Y, Lepine JP, et al. The epidemiology of traumatic event exposure worldwide: results from the world mental health survey consortium. Psychol Med. 2016;46(2):327–43. https://doi.org/10.1017/S0033291715001981.
5. Blevins CA, Weathers FW, Davis MT, Witte TK, Domino JL. The posttraumatic stress disorder checklist for DSM-5 (PCL-5): Development and Initial Psychometric Evaluation. J Trauma Stress. 2015;28(6):489–98. https://doi.org/10.1002/jts.22059.
6. Bockhop F, Zeldovich M, Cunitz K, Van Praag D, van der Vlegel M, Beissbarth T, Hagmayer Y, von Steinbuechel N, CENTER-TBI participants and investigators. Measurement invariance of six language versions of the post-traumatic stress disorder checklist for DSM-5 in civilians after traumatic brain injury. Sci Rep. 2022;12(1):16571. https://doi.org/10.1038/s41598-022-20170-2.
7. Bradley R, Greene J, Russ E, Dutra L, Westen D. A multidimensional meta-analysis of psychotherapy for PTSD.Am J Psychiatry. 2005;162(2):214-227. https://doi.org/10.1176/appi.ajp.162.2.214.
8. Center for Substance Abuse Treatment. (2014). Trauma-informed care in behavioral health services (Treatment Improvement Protocol [TIP] Series No. 57, Chapter 3: Understanding the impact of trauma). Substance Abuse and Mental Health Services Administration. https://www.ncbi.nlm.nih.gov/books/NBK207191/
9. Ehlers A, Gene-Cos N, Perrin S. Low recognition of posttraumatic stress disorder in primary care. Lond J Prim Care. 2009;2:36–42. https://doi.org/10.1080/17571472.2009.11493255.
10. Foa EB, Hembree EA, Rothbaum BO, Rauch SAM. Prolonged exposure therapy for PTSD: Emotional processing of traumatic experiences: Therapist guide (2nd ed.). Oxford University Press. 2019. https://doi.org/10.1093/med-psych/9780190926939.001.0001.
11. Forkus SR, Raudales AM, Rafiuddin HS, Weiss NH, Messman BA, Contractor AA. The posttraumatic stress disorder (PTSD) checklist for DSM-5: a systematic review of existing psychometric evidence. Clin Psychol. 2023;30(1):110–21. https://doi.org/10.1037/cps0000111.
12. Greene T, Neria Y, Gross R. Prevalence, detection and correlates of PTSD in the primary care setting: a systematic review. J Clin Psychol Med Settings. 2016;23(2):160–80. https://doi.org/10.1007/s10880-016-9455-3.
13. Hall BJ, Yip PSY, Garabiles MR, Lao CK, Chan EWW, Marx BP. Psychometric validation of the PTSD Checklist-5 among female Filipino migrant workers. Eur J Psychotraumatol. 2019;10(1):1571378. https://doi.org/10.1080/20008198.2019.1571378.
14. Harrington T. The clinician-administered PTSD scale for children and adolescents: a validation study. Dissertation Abstracts Int: Sect B: Sci Eng. n.d.;69(8-B):5028.
15. Hollifield M, Hsiao AF, Smith T, Calloway T, Jovanovic T, Smith B, Carrick K, Norrholm SD, Munoz A, Alpert R, Caicedo B, Frousakis N, Cocozza K. Acupuncture for combat-related posttraumatic stress disorder: a randomized clinical trial. JAMA Psychiatry. 2024;81(6):545–54. https://doi.org/10.1001/jamapsychiatry.2023.5651.
16. Huang RW, Shen T, Ge LM, Cao L, Luo JF, Wu SY. Psychometric properties of the Chinese version of the primary care post-traumatic stress disorder Screen-5 for medical staff exposed

to the COVID-19 pandemic. Psychol Res Behav Manag. 2021;14:1371–8. https://doi.org/10.2147/PRBM.S329380.
17. Ibrahim H, Ertl V, Catani C, Ismail AA, Neuner F. The validity of posttraumatic stress disorder checklist for DSM-5 (PCL-5) as screening instrument with Kurdish and Arab displaced populations living in the Kurdistan region of Iraq. BMC Psychiatry. 2018;18(1):259. https://doi.org/10.1186/s12888-018-1839-z.
18. Johnson DR, Lubin H. Principles and techniques of trauma-centered psychotherapy. American Psychiatric Publishing; 2015.
19. Jones K, Boschen M, Devilly G, Vogler J, Flowers H, Winkleman C, Wullschleger M. Risk and protective factors that predict posttraumatic stress disorder after traumatic injury: a systematic review. Health Sci Rev. 2024;10:100147. https://doi.org/10.1016/j.hsr.2023.100147.
20. Kaplan J, Somohano VC, Zaccari B, O'Neil ME. Randomized controlled trials of mind-body interventions for posttraumatic stress disorder: a systematic review. Front Psychol. 2024;14:1219296. https://doi.org/10.3389/fpsyg.2023.1219296.
21. Kouki N, Bourgou S, Rezgui H, Naffeti A, Hamdoun M, Belhadj A. Clinician-Administered PTSD Scale for DSM-5, child and adolescent version: A transcultural validation. Eur Psychiatry. 2023;66(Suppl 1):S737. https://doi.org/10.1192/j.eurpsy.2023.1548.
22. Kube T, Elssner AC, Herzog P. The relationship between multiple traumatic events and the severity of posttraumatic stress disorder symptoms – evidence for a cognitive link. Eur J Psychotraumatol. 2023;14(1):2165025. https://doi-org.ezproxy.cul.columbia.edu/10.1080/20008066.2023.2165025
23. Lerner MJ, Miller DT. Just world research and the attribution process: looking back and ahead. Psychol Bull. 1978;85(5):1030–51. https://doi-org.ezproxy.cul.columbia.edu/10.1037/0033-2909.85.5.1030
24. Libby DJ, Pilver CE, Desai R. Complementary and alternative medicine use among individuals with posttraumatic stress disorder. Psychol Trauma Theory Res Pract Policy. 2013;5(3):277–85. https://doi.org/10.1037/a0027082.
25. Liebschutz J, Saitz R, Brower V, Keane TM, Lloyd-Travaglini C, Averbuch T, Samet JH. PTSD in urban primary care: high prevalence and low physician recognition. J Gen Intern Med. 2007;22(6):719–26. https://doi.org/10.1007/s11606-007-0161-0.
26. Littleton HL. The impact of social support and negative disclosure reactions on sexual assault victims: a cross-sectional and longitudinal investigation. J Trauma Dissociation. 2010;11(2):210–27. https://doi-org.ezproxy.cul.columbia.edu/10.1080/15299730903502946
27. Liu P, Wang L, Cao C, Wang R, Zhang J, Zhang B, Wu Q, Zhang H, Zhao Z, Fan G, Elhai JD. The underlying dimensions of DSM-5 posttraumatic stress disorder symptoms in an epidemiological sample of Chinese earthquake survivors. J Anxiety Disord. 2014;28(4):345–51. https://doi.org/10.1016/j.janxdis.2014.03.008.
28. Liu Q, Zhu J, Zhang W. The efficacy of mindfulness-based stress reduction intervention 3 for post-traumatic stress disorder (PTSD) symptoms in patients with PTSD: a meta-analysis of four randomized controlled trials. Stress Health. 2022;38(4):626–36. https://doi.org/10.1002/smi.3138.
29. Monson CM, Shnaider P. Treating PTSD With Cognitive-Behavioral Therapies: Interventions That Work. Washington, DC: American Psychological Association; 2014.
30. Öst LG, Enebrink P, Finnes A, et al. Cognitive behavior therapy for adult post-traumatic stress disorder in routine clinical care: A systematic review and meta-analysis. Behav Res Ther. 2023;166:104323. https://doi.org/10.1016/j.brat.2023.104323.
31. Pacella ML, Hruska B, Delahanty DL. The physical health consequences of PTSD and PTSD symptoms: a meta-analytic review. J Anxiety Disord. 2013;27(1):33–46. https://doi.org/10.1016/j.janxdis.2012.08.004.
32. Prins A, Bovin MJ, Kimerling R, Kaloupek DG, Marx BP, Pless Kaiser A, Schnurr PP. The primary care PTSD screen for DSM-5 (PC-PTSD-5): development and evaluation within a veteran primary care sample. J Gen Intern Med. 2015; https://doi.org/10.1007/s11606-016-3703-5.

33. Pynoos RS, Weathers FW, Steinberg AM, Marx BP, Layne CM, Kaloupek DG, Schnurr PP, Keane TM, Blake DD, Newman E, Nader KO, Kriegler JA. Clinician-administered PTSD scale for DSM-5 – Child/adolescent version. [Assessment]. Psychol Assess. 2015. Available from the National Center for PTSD at www.PTSD.va.gov.
34. Resick PA, Monson CM, Chard KM. Cognitive Processing Therapy for PTSD: A Comprehensive Manual. New York, NY: Guilford Press; 2016.
35. Saltzman KM, Weems CF, Carrion VG. IQ and posttraumatic stress symptoms in children exposed to interpersonal violence. Child Psychiatry Hum Dev. 2006;36(3):261–72. https://doi.org/10.1007/s10578-005-0002-5.
36. Tang X, Lin S, Fang D, Lin B, Yao L, Wang L, Xu Q, Lu L, Xu N. Efficacy and underlying mechanisms of acupuncture therapy for PTSD: evidence from animal and clinical studies. Front Behav Neurosci. 2023;17:1163718. https://doi.org/10.3389/fnbeh.2023.1163718.
37. Tedeschi RG, Calhoun LG. The posttraumatic growth inventory: measuring the positive legacy of trauma. J Trauma Stress. 1996;9(3):455–71. https://doi.org/10.1007/BF02103658.
38. U.S. Department of Veterans Affairs. PTSD checklist for DSM-5 (PCL-5). National Center for PTSD; n.d.. https://www.PTSD.va.gov/professional/assessment/adult-sr/PTSD-checklist.asp
39. van de Kamp MM, Scheffers M, Emck C, Fokker TJ, Hatzmann J, Cuijpers P, Beek PJ. Body- and movement-oriented interventions for posttraumatic stress disorder: an updated systematic review and meta-analysis. J Trauma Stress. 2023;36(5):835–48. https://doi.org/10.1002/jts.22968.
40. Waszczuk MA, Li X, Bromet EJ, Gonzalez A, Zvolensky MJ, Ruggero C, et al. Pathway from PTSD to respiratory health: longitudinal evidence from a psychosocial intervention. Health Psychol. 2017;36(5):429–37. https://doi.org/10.1037/hea0000455.
41. Weathers FW, Litz BT, Keane TM, Palmieri PA, Marx BP, Schnurr PP. The PTSD checklist for DSM-5 (PCL-5). 2013. Scale available from the National Center for PTSD at https://www.ptsd.va.gov.
42. Zayfert C, DeViva J. Avoiding treatment failures in PTSD. In: Otto MW, Hofmann SG, editors. Avoiding treatment failures in the anxiety disorders. Springer; 2009. p. 147–69.

Chapter 5
Insomnia

Nataliya Pilipenko, Krishna M. Desai, and Aury Garcia

Case Vignette

Mr. H is a 71-year-old man with a history of hypertension, rheumatoid arthritis, and asthma. He is presenting for evaluation of long-standing sleep difficulties.

Mr. H: *I've had a really hard time falling asleep. I wake up in the middle of the night and can't get back to sleep. I only sleep three to four hours at night. It started ten years ago but it's been worse over the last year. At first, I thought it was stress, and it happened only occasionally, but since last year it happens four or five nights a week.*

Dr. K: *And when you first go to bed, how long does it take you to fall asleep?*

Mr. H: *Usually more than an hour. I'll go to bed around 10:30 pm, but I just lie there staring at the ceiling.*

Dr. K: *Are you napping during the day to catch up on sleep?*

N. Pilipenko (✉)
Center for Family and Community Medicine, Department of Medicine, Columbia University Irving Medical Center/New York Presbyterian Hospital, New York, NY, USA

Department of Psychiatry, Columbia University Irving Medical Center, New York, NY, USA
e-mail: np2615@cumc.columbia.edu

K. M. Desai
Center for Family and Community Medicine, Department of Medicine, Columbia University Irving Medical Center/New York Presbyterian Hospital, New York, NY, USA

Center for Neuroinflammatory and Somatic Disorders, Department of Psychiatry, Columbia University Irving Medical Center, New York, NY, USA

A. Garcia
Center for Family and Community Medicine, Department of Medicine, Columbia University Irving Medical Center/New York Presbyterian Hospital, New York, NY, USA

N. Pilipenko, K. M. Desai (eds.), *8 Conditions Primary Care Clinicians Dread to Treat*, https://doi.org/10.1007/978-3-032-12819-5_5

Mr. H: *Not really. I take care of my grandkids and by the afternoon I'm so tired. I'm always running on low*

Dr. K: *It sounds like this has been ongoing for a while and problems with sleep are really affecting your daily life. When you go to bed, are you giving yourself enough time to sleep?*

Mr. H: *Yes, I am in bed by 10:30 pm and don't get up until about 8 am. I try to wind down in the evening, no coffee, no tv, no phone but my brain just won't stop going.*

Dr. K: *And what are your goals for sleep?*

Mr. H: *I want to go to bed and fall asleep within 30 minutes or so, sleep for the rest of the night, get up in the morning, and go about doing my business. Maybe seven to eight hours of sleep. Does this seem reasonable to you?*

Dr. K: *Yes, these are realistic goals. Can I tell you about my "first line" recommendations for patients who experience similar sleep problems?*

Diagnosis: Brief Description

Per DSM-5-TR [1] **insomnia** disorder is characterized by dissatisfaction with sleep quantity or quality concerning: sleep initiation, sleep maintenance, or early morning awakening. Sleep problems must be present at least three nights per week for at least three months and lead to distress and/or functional impairment. Etiological effects of relevant substances (e.g. caffeine), **medication**s (e.g., beta blockers, steroids) and medical conditions (e.g. restless leg syndrome) must be ruled out. Please refer to DSM-5-TR [1] for information pertaining to the differential diagnostic considerations.

Physicians should be familiar with the following terms:

1. Sleep latency (SL): time needed to fall asleep. Prolonged SL is >20–30 min [[1], p. 411].
2. Early morning awakenings: awakening at least 1 hour before scheduled wake up time and after less than 6.5 hours of sleep [1, p. 411].
3. Sleep efficiency (SE): Is calculated by dividing a patient's Total Sleep Time by Time In Bed (in minutes) and multiplying by 100. SE is the key metric for sleep improvement **tracking**. Typically, goal SE is >80–85%.

Prevalence, Risk Factors, and Disparities

Prevalence of **insomnia** in the general U.S., population ranges from 4–22% [1] while in primary care (PC) it is 20–40% [2]. Psychiatric and medical comorbidities are common yet overlooked cause and/or exacerbating factors [3, 25].

Increased rates of **insomnia** severity in older age appear to be driven by accumulating number of medical conditions, however, for reasons that are not well understood this "trend appears more pronounced among Hispanic older adults than in non-Hispanic whites" [17]. Furthermore, negative social factors (also known as social vulnerability) can play a role in **insomnia** severity.

Symptom Assessment Tools

Table 5.1 presents three common screening tools: **Insomnia** Severity Index (ISI, [20]), Athens **Insomnia** Scale (AIS, [27]) and Pittsburgh Sleep Quality Index (PSQI, [6]). While AIS assesses the severity of **insomnia** symptoms using International Classification of Diseases (ICD-10) diagnostic criteria, both ISI and PSQI focus on subjective sleep quality and daytime functioning. Additionally, PSQI assesses patient's use of sleeping medication. Although all three instruments are copyrighted, they are freely accessible with a simple registration process.

Table 5.1 Insomnia disorder screening tools

Screener name	Items #	Rating scale scoring	Cut offs	Assessment timeline	Availability	Psychometric properties	Non-English versions available?
Insomnia Severity Index (ISI)	7 [20]	5-point likert [20] 0 = none/very satisfied/not at all interfering/not at all noticeable/not at all 4 = very/very dissatisfied/very much interfering/very much noticeable/very much	0–7 = no clinically significant insomnia [20] 8–14 = subthreshold insomnia 15–21 = clinical insomnia (moderate severity) 22–28 = clinical insomnia (severe)	2 weeks [20]	Copyrighted [20]	Internal consistency [20] (α = .90–.91) Score = 10 showed [20] sensitivity = 86.1% Specificity = 87.7% for detecting insomnia	Arabic [29], Chinese [26], Spanish [10]

Athens Insomnia Scale (AIS)	8 [27]	4-point likert [27] 0 = no problem/ not earlier/ sufficient/ satisfactory/ normal/none to 3 = very delayed/ serious problem/ much earlier/ very insufficient/ very unsatisfied/ very decreased/ intense	0–5 = lower normal daytime [27] sleepiness 6–10 = higher normal daytime sleepiness 11–12 = mild excessive daytime sleepiness 13–15 = moderate excessive daytime sleepiness 16–24 = severe excessive daytime sleepiness Cutoff score of 6 [28] distinguished between insomnia and patients without insomnia in 90% of cases	1 month [27]	Copyrighted [27]	Internal consistency [27] (α = .87–.89) Test-retest reliability [27] = .88–.89	Arabic [13], Chinese [31], Spanish [12]
Pittsburgh Sleep Quality Index (PSQI)	10 [6]	Combination of open-ended questions and likert scales [6] Item 10 not scored, used for clinical purposes 0 = not during the past month to 3 = three or more times a week	Score of 5 correctly [6] identified 88.5% of patient group in validation study	1 month [6]	Copyrighted [6]	Internal reliability [6] (α = .83) Test–retest reliability = .85 Sensitivity = 89.6%, and specificity = 86.5%	Arabic (Tunisia) [5], Chinese [35], Spanish [15]

Non-pharmacological Conceptualization: What to Say to the Patient?

Message #1: Sleep Concerns Must Be Approached Holistically

Adequate sleep is important for overall physical and psychological health. In general, adults between ages of 18 and 64 are recommended to sleep seven to nine hours, while adults over the age of 65 are recommended to sleep seven to eight hours [21].

Poor sleep can result from many physical and mental health issues, oftentimes, several such issues are negatively affecting sleep at the same time. For example, depression can lead to difficulty falling asleep, poor quality of sleep, or early morning awakenings, while chronic pain may cause frequent "tossing and turning." Excess weight is a strong risk factor for obstructive sleep apnea (OSA) which can lead to morning headaches and daytime fatigue. To improve sleep, treatment strategies should address these contributing factors. Some of these problems can be managed well with **medication**s, others (like chronic pain, for example) require a more comprehensive, whole person approach, because no **medication** can cure these conditions.

Regardless of the underlying causes of poor sleep, several well established, non-**medication** strategies are available. These strategies are considered "first line" treatments, meaning that they are the most effective techniques that are currently developed for improving sleep.

Why? Good sleep is linked to improved cardiovascular health, mental health, cognition, memory consolidation, immunity, reproductive health, and hormone regulation [4]. However, a wide range of medical conditions are associated with sleep disruption. Specifically: cardiac (congestive heart failure, arrhythmias), pulmonary (asthma, COPD) gastrointestinal (GERD, hepatic encephalopathy), musculoskeletal (arthritis, fibromyalgia), neurologic (dementia, epilepsy, migraines/headaches, neurodegenerative disorders), endocrine (hyperthyroidism, menopause), dermatologic (pruritic skin conditions), urologic (benign prostatic hypertrophy, overactive bladder) [30]. Furthermore, common psychiatric conditions such as Major Depressive Disorder and Generalized Anxiety Disorder encompass sleep-related symptoms [1].

As sleep concerns related to medical and psychiatric conditions can be potentially ameliorated by improved control of these underlying conditions, it is important to ensure that the patient understands the link between their management and improved sleep. Thus, when appropriate, discussion of poor sleep can be framed within the context of overall care engagement, rather than treated as a separate symptom.

However, regardless of the etiology, behavioral factors often play a significant role in occurrence, maintenance, and exacerbation of **insomnia** and behavioral interventions are the first line for treatment [19].

Message #2: Accurate Expectations Are Key

Many patients are interested in sleep **medication**s. However, there are no **medications** that are recommended beyond five weeks of use. Unfortunately, currently available **medication**s are unable to radically increase sleep duration or its quality long-term. Some **medication**s can be unsafe or make sleep problems worse over time. Furthermore, patients also buy **medication**s (e.g. ZzzQuil, benadryl), herbs (e.g. valerian) or supplements (e.g. melatonin) to improve sleep. However, none of these are recommended for long-term sleep problems and some can make **insomnia** even harder to treat (See Resources for patient education materials).

Current medical guidelines state that all patients suffering from **insomnia** start treatment by addressing their sleep behaviors, because these (behavioral) interventions are both safe and effective. However, it is important that a good faith effort to change behavioral patterns is made—techniques cannot work unless these are used consistently. If behavioral interventions are not fully addressing the sleep concern, then **medication**s can be discussed.

Why? Chronic **insomnia** management guidelines by the American College of Physicians [23], recommend cognitive behavioral interventions as first line of **insomnia** treatment while use of pharmacotherapy should be limited in time and involve discussion about risks, harms, and costs. Moreover, these guidelines emphasize that the Food and Drug Administration approves pharmacotherapy for **insomnia** for up to four to five weeks and treatment should be evaluated further if **insomnia** symptoms do not remit within seven to ten days [22]. Finally, American Academy of Sleep Medicine [24] advises against use of diphenhydramine, tryptophan, melatonin, valerian for **insomnia,** while commonly prescribed trazodone is also not recommended for **insomnia** treatment.

Next section of the Vignette illustrates questions assessing **medication**-related knowledge, risks, and long-term **insomnia** management plans. These questions can guide patient-physician discussion in constructive key.

Case Vignette—Continued

Mr. H: *I wanted to talk to you about* ***medication****s for my sleep problem. I just want to take something that will let me sleep right away. One of my friends told me about a medicine called [names* ***medication*** *X, a benzodiazepine]. Can you just send that to the pharmacy for me?*

Dr. K: *Once you start* ***medication****s, what changes do you expect to see?*

Mr. H: *I am hoping these will help me start to sleep normally again.*

Dr. K: *From what we know,* ***medication****s at best can provide a small benefit when used for less than four to five weeks when there are short-term sleeping issues.* [Review Message #2] *What do you understand about the potential risks of [medication X]?*

Mr. H: *I have not heard about any risks. Are there any I should know about? It's just that I am in so much pain at night because of my rheumatoid arthritis. I just want to take something that will knock me out until the next day.*

Dr. K: [Review risks of **medications**] *Since your pain is making it harder to sleep, let's talk about how to manage your pain too.* (Please see Chapter #6—Chronic pain). *If* ***medications*** *don't help with sleep, are there any alternatives you can think of?*

Mr. H: *I am kind of at a loss. I am hoping you will point me in the right direction to get my sleep back on track.*

Dr. K: *It is important to approach sleep difficulties from multiple angles. If you are okay with it, I would like to talk to you about all your options. We should review the different types of* ***medications*** *available including the risks and benefits. In addition, it is also very important to consider some potential changes in behavior that can help improve your sleep over the long run.*

Mr. H: *How can we do that?*

Dr. K: *We need to start by getting a better understanding of how you sleep; what makes your sleep better and worse. This can be hard to notice if you are not recording specifics daily. I recommend that all patients with* ***insomnia*** *track their sleep every day for two weeks. I can give you a pen and paper diary or an app option for* ***tracking****.*

Mr. H: *This sounds like it may be helpful.*

Dr. K: *We will review this information when you come back and look for patterns. I will also be able to give you recommendations which are specific for addressing your unique sleep patterns. What do you think about* ***tracking*** *for two weeks?*

Mr. H: *Okay. Give me a paper diary then. I will give it a go.*

Non-pharmacological Treatment Options: What Can Be Done?

Brief behavioral interventions can be highly effective for insomnia management and can be incorporated within a standard PC visit. Key to success, however, lies in providing clear instructions and reviewing results of the initial sleep modification efforts in order to spotlight and address contributing factors and behaviors.

1. **Instruct Patient to Engage in Sleep Tracking**

As the first step, it is important for patients to track sleep for at least two weeks (and up to two months in perimenopausal and menopausal women). **Tracking** helps patients and physicians understand sleep patterns and implicated behavioral factors. Although it may seem daunting to many patients, this short-term strategy provides crucial information to guide behavioral interventions. Continuity of **tracking** is important—patients should be explicitly asked to track on both good and bad sleep days. Pen-and-paper as well as app-based options are available (See Resources).

Why? Subjective accounts of sleep difficulties can be unreliable; thus, **tracking** offers a critical tool for improved understanding of the sleep concerns as well as treatment planning.

Several sleep patterns may contribute to poor sleep and should be monitored for, when **tracking** is reviewed:

A. *Significant Variability in Total Sleep Time (TST)*

Patients may be "sleeping in" certain days (typically weekends) or taking prolonged daytime naps. Although such behaviors often result from desire to "catch up" on sleep they lead to trouble falling asleep in the evening thus shortening the next day's TST and perpetuating the **insomnia** cycle. This problem may be particularly salient for patients who have strict wake up time the following day (e.g. patients who wake up early for work during the weekdays).

B. *Contrariety Between TST and Desired Wake up Time*

Some patients may complain of early morning awakening, however review of bedtime may indicate that wake-up time is in fact consistent with sleep expectations and norms. For example, a patient going to sleep at 8 pm will wake up at 4 am after 8 hours of sleep. This information should be carefully reviewed and sleep patterns should explained to the patient.

2. **Focus on Sleep Consolidation**

To increase the duration of sleep, many patients attempt to increase time in bed. For example, going to bed early (or when not feeling sleepy), staying in bed at night or during the day despite being unable to sleep, and/or taking daytime naps. In extreme cases, patients may remain in bed and/or laying down throughout most of the day. Although such strategies aim to increase sleep opportunities, they set up a long-standing pattern of poor sleep via:

A. *Associative Learning*

Through the process of classical conditioning, the patient's bed becomes associated with being awake rather than being asleep, thus making it more difficult to fall asleep.

B. *Lack of Tiredness*

Low levels of daytime activities combined with protracted time in bed, lead to low levels of tiredness, thus the patient is simply not yet sleepy at bedtime. Similarly, protracted daytime naps or late awakenings (e.g. sleeping in on the weekends), lead to low evening tiredness, delay in falling asleep and subsequent fatigue the following morning. Thus, it is less important the patients keep the same bedtime, but it is central that wake up time is kept (approximately) the same throughout the week.

To manage these behaviors, *Sleep Efficiency (SE)* (see Diagnosis: Brief Description section) should be calculated and discussed upon the review of **tracking**. Many apps automatically calculate this metric. Patients should be informed that achieving SE optimization is the first step to addressing insomnia. Once the SE goal is achieved (typically set at 80–85%) total sleep time can be gradually increased. Specifically, patients can increase time in bed by 15 min every two weeks, as long as the SE % is maintained. Typically, this means going to bed 15 min earlier than currently maintained bedtime.

3. **Ask Patients to Avoid All Forms of Visual Stimulation in Bed**
Although many patients are asked to "avoid screen time" few are appraised to the reasons why this behavior is contraindicated. The following script outlines the rationale behind this recommendation:

> Our sleep is very strongly affected by light exposure. Specifically, we wake up in response to light shining on our eyelids which stimulates hormones that wake us up. When we read/watch tv/use phone or tablet, the light can be very strong, and it goes directly through our pupil (the small black hole right in the middle), stimulating the brain cells and preventing them from powering down. So, using reading or scrolling to help with falling asleep, on a physiological level is akin to putting out fire with gasoline.

Psychotherapy Effectiveness: Insomnia

APA's Society of Clinical Psychology (n.d) lists cognitive behavioral therapy (CBT) as well as its subcomponents (stimulus control, sleep restriction, relaxation training, and paradoxical intention) as having strong research support, while biofeedback for **insomnia** is noted to have modest research support.

Unlike other EBPs, psychotherapy protocols for **insomnia** are characterized by significant variability in methodologies (see van Straten et al. [32] for further discussion). However, overall, both full cognitive behavioral therapy (CBT) protocol for **insomnia** and its sub-parts are associated with **insomnia** improvement. Specifically, improvements are noted for sleep efficiency ($g = 0.71$), wake after sleep onset ($g = 0.63$) and sleep onset latency ($g = 0.57$), and number of awakenings ($g = 0.29$) and sleep quality ($g = 0.40$).

Finally, there is a growing body of research supporting delivery of internet-based interventions. Specifically, 8-week RCT examining CBTi intervention for somatic symptom distress, noted significant improvements both in SSD measures as well as measures of depression, anxiety, illness worries, functional impairment, with over 70% completion rate and 90% of participants reporting satisfaction [14].

Table 5.2 outlines CBT-based instructions for patients which, when followed concurrently and consistently, lead to significant improvement in **insomnia** symptoms.

Table 5.2 Sleep improvement recommendation

Only go to bed when feeling tired (no need for set bedtime)	Avoid daytime naps. If taking a nap seems necessary, limit it to 30 min (set an alarm)
If unable to fall asleep within 20 min, leave the bed and engage in relaxing, non-visual activity (e.g. listening to music, sound of nature). Avoid anything that is stimulating—cleaning, etc. Only return to bed when feeling sleepy	Engage in daytime activities (these do not need to be outside of home; however, lack of mental and/or physical stimulation will contribute to poor sleep)
Keep wake up time approximately the same throughout the week	Bed is only for sex and sleep

Integrative Medicine Interventions and Techniques

Integrative Medicine (IM) therapies can be incorporated as adjunctive strategies in the management of **insomnia**. These interventions can be safely combined for potentially additive therapeutic effect.

Lifestyle Medicine (LM)

Negative impact of behaviors on sleep such as sedentary lifestyle, increased screen time, diets high in processed foods and sugars, substance misuse, high levels of stress are well documented in literature and frequently observed in clinical practice. A systematic review and metanalysis demonstrated positive impact of LM intervention on improving sleep quality ($d = 1.02$, 95% *CI* [−1.37, −0.67]). Furthermore, individuals with a clinical level of sleep disturbance had a larger effect size than those with sub-clinical levels of sleep disturbance ($d = -0.57$, 95% *CI* [−0.82, −0.32]) [34].

Mind-Body Interventions (MBI)

Meditative movement based **mind-body** interventions such as yoga and Tai Chi significantly improve sleep efficiency *(d = 1.22, 95% CI [0.13, 2.32])* and significantly reduce severity of sleep problem (d = −0.86, 95% CI [−1.59, −0.13] [9].

Herbs, Botanicals, and Supplements

A variety of herbs, botanicals, and supplements (HBS), including melatonin, valerian (*Valeriana officinalis*), chamomile (*Matricaria recutita*), ashwagandha (*Withania somnifera*), passionflower (*Passiflora incarnata*), skullcap (*Scutellaria lateriflora*), and hops (*Humulus lupulus*) are used by patients to address sleep concerns. Except for melatonin, however, high-quality evidence is lacking to recommend most of these products.

Melatonin

Melatonin is widely available over the counter in a wide variety of doses and formulations, however systematic reviews and meta-analyses of RCTs show it only produces modest reduction in sleep onset latency and increases in total sleep time compared to placebo [11]. It does have a favorable safety profile and can be recommended if patients are very interested in trying it. A more recent meta-analysis from 2024 suggested that a 4 mg dose administered approximately 3 h before the desired bedtime may optimize efficacy [7]. Many studies have used lower doses and patients are often recommended to use lower doses immediately before bedtime which may be less effective. It needs to be noted however, that current American Academy of Sleep Medicine (AASM, [24]) do not recommend melatonin for long-term treatment.

Micronutrient Deficiencies

Micronutrient deficiencies can also contribute to sleep disturbances. Specifically, low levels of iron, B vitamins, zinc, calcium, vitamin K, magnesium, and vitamin D are linked to impaired sleep quality [16, 18, 36]. When dietary patterns, **medication** use, or comorbid conditions indicate increased risk of micronutrient deficiencies, physicians should order targeted laboratory assessments (e.g., ferritin, serum magnesium, 25-hydroxy-vitamin D) and correct any confirmed deficiencies with standard dosing regimens. Patients can also be referred to dieticians for counseling and optimizing nutritional intake which is also necessary for overall health.

Clinical Pearls

- Brief screeners (**Insomnia** Severity Index (ISI), Athens **Insomnia** Scale (AIS) and Pittsburgh Sleep Quality Index can assist with prompt assessment of **insomnia** symptoms and support the diagnosis
- A holistic approach to **insomnia** care (including management of implicated comorbidities) is key.
- Explicitly address patient's treatment expectations, including expectation for long-term pharmacotherapy
- Behavioral strategies are "first line" interventions for **insomnia** but require consistent engagement and patient's active participation
- Use **tracking** to identify patterns contributing to **insomnia**. Once identify, instruct patient to change these as appropriate
- Focus on behavioral antecedents and maintaining factors of sleep

Frequently Asked Questions

Question 1: *I am already avoiding caffeine and sleeping in a dark room. Why is my sleep not improving?*

Answer: Despite its popularity, sleep hygiene interventions have demonstrated only limited utility for **insomnia** [33]. However, changing sleep behaviors, particularly avoiding time in bed when not sleeping, avoiding screentime, and inconsistent sleep schedules can lead to significant sleep improvement (for further details see Desai et al. [8]).

Question 2: *I am going to bed at the same time every day, why is my sleep not improving?*

Answer: It is more important to keep waking up the same, going to bed when not feeling sleepy can contribute to poor sleep. Specifically, the brain learns to associate being in bed with not being asleep, making it harder to fall asleep when needed.

Question 3: *I have been having trouble sleeping for years and I tried so many things already. Why can't I get a pill to make my sleep better?*

Answer: Unfortunately, no **medication** can safely be used long term and no **medication** greatly increases sleep duration or quality. Many patients find themselves quickly frustrated by behavioral intervention and quickly return to using phone in bed/watching tv/sleeping in or staying in bed when not sleeping. What is important to remember is that behavioral techniques require consistent application and time. If you are only using them some days and not others, they are unlikely to help. What I recommend is that you commit to following all behavioral recommendations for about 4 weeks while **tracking** your sleep. We can review together and try to solve problems if any sleep concerns remain after that point.

Resources

Source	Description	Link
Tracking Resources		
Insomnia Coach App	Free app which includes tracking diary as well as multiple helpful tips for sleep improvement. Available for iOS and Android	https://www.ptsd.va.gov/appvid/mobile/insomnia_coach.asp
National Heart Lung and Blood Institute	Printable sleep diary—1 page	https://www.nhlbi.nih.gov/resources/sleep-diary
National Sleep Foundation	Printable sleep diary—2 pages	https://pa-foundation.org/wp-content/uploads/NSF-Sleep-Diary.pdf
Office of Developmental Primary Care, University of California, San Francisco	Printable sleep diary in Spanish—2 pages	https://odpc.ucsf.edu/sites/odpc.ucsf.edu/libraries/pdf.js/web/viewer.html?file=https%3A%2F%2Fodpc.ucsf.edu%2Fsites%2Fodpc.ucsf.edu%2Ffiles%2Fdocuments%2F19.%2520Sleep%2520Log-SPANISH.pdf
Relaxation Apps to Support Sleep		
Headspace	Free app provides several audio meditations	https://nyc988.cityofnewyork.us/apps/headspace/
Sanvello	Free app provides several audio meditations. Available Spanish text	https://nyc988.cityofnewyork.us/apps/sanvello/

(continued)

Source	Description	Link
RainRain	Free app with sounds of rain. Available for iOS and Android	https://www.rainrainapp.com/
Patient Education Resources		
American Academy of Sleep Medicine (AASM)	Brief patient guide to medications which are recommended for chronic insomnia	https://aasm.org/wp-content/uploads/2019/11/Pharma-Insomnia-Patient-Guide.pdf
American Academy of Sleep Medicine (AASM)	Brief patient guide to medications which are recommended for chronic insomnia—Spanish	https://aasm.org/wp-content/uploads/2020/06/Pharma-Insomnia-Patient-Guide-Spanish.pdf
American Academy of Sleep Medicine (AASM)	A patient's guide to understanding Behavioral and Psychological Treatments for Chronic Insomnia Disorder in Adults	https://aasm.org/wp-content/uploads/2021/08/Behavioral-and-Psychological-Treatments-for-Insomnia-Patient-Guide.pdf
American Psychological Association, Division of Clinical Psychology (12)	Offers review (including evaluation of the strength of supporting evidence) for various insomnia psychotherapies Click on each treatment to learn more. When available, information about treatment manuals and bibliotherapy is provided	https://div12.org/treatments/?_sfm_related_diagnosis=8146
Digital Therapeutics		
Somryst	FDA- approved app, delivers 9 week cognitive behavioral therapy for insomnia. Requires prescription	https://dtxalliance.org/products/somryst/
Sleepio	Fully automated digital sleep improvement program based on Cognitive Behavioral Therapy (CBT) Should be used under supervision of a healthcare professional	https://info.sleepio.com/suitability#:~:text=Sleepio%20is%20a%20digital%20therapeutic,supervision%20of%20a%20healthcare%20professional

Case Vignette—Conclusion

Mr. H. returns to discuss treatment options for insomnia after **tracking** his sleep pattern for the past two weeks. His log is presented above. Dr. K reviews the log. (Table 5.3).

Dr. K: *Thank you for completing the tracking. Did you have any problems doing so?*

Mr. H. *It was ok. The app did not work for me so I used pen and paper diary. I just hope this can help.*

Dr. K: [looking at the tracking data]. *Can I tell you what stands out to me right away?*

Mr. H: *Tell me.*

Dr. K: *It looks like you are in bed two hours before falling asleep.*

Mr. H: *That's right, I feel tired but can't fall asleep yet.*

Dr. K.: *Your logic makes perfect sense to me. However staying in bed when not sleeping can make it harder to fall asleep since your brain learns that bed is for being awake. I would suggest going to bed only when you are planning to sleep.*

Mr. H: *That makes sense. I tend to lay in the bed even if I am just hanging out watching TV or talking on the phone.*

Dr. K: [Discusses: Non-pharmacological Treatment Options: What can be done? Point #3].

Mr. H: *It sounds like I should go to bed when I'm sleepy and try to avoid screens. What do I do if I cannot fall asleep right away?*

Dr. K: *If you can't fall asleep within 20 minutes, get out of bed and do something calming like listening to relaxing music.*

Mr. H: *That makes a lot of sense? What else do you see as a problem?*

Dr. K: *On the days you wake up very early, around 6:30 am, it looks like you fall asleep early as well and wake up sooner than expected, in the middle of the night.*

Mr. H: *Yeah, that tends to happen and then I feel like I am in a vicious cycle that makes my sleep even worse.*

Dr. K: *In these situations, it may help to set a more consistent time to go to bed and wake up. You can also consider a scheduled 30-minute nap during the day to get back on track.*

Mr. H: *I will try these tips and let you know if my sleep gets better.*

Table 5.3 Mr. H sleep diary

Day of the week	Bedtime	Sleep time	Wake up time	Awake in bed before falling asleep again	Out of bed	Sleep efficiency	Comments
Monday	10:30 pm	12:00 am	2:00 am	60 min	8:30 am	450/600 × 100 = 75%	
Tuesday	10:30 pm	11:30 pm	3:00 am	90 min	8:30 am	450/600 × 100 = 75%	
Wednesday	10:30 pm	12:00 am	2:00 am	60 min	6:30 am	450/480 × 100 = 93.75%	Woke up early to take care of grandkids
Thursday	9:00 pm	10:30 am	3:00 am	180 min	9:30 am	450/750 × 100 = 60%	
Friday	7:00 pm	Unknown	2:00 am	Unknown	6:30 am	420/690 × 100 = 61%	Too tired, fell asleep without meaning to while watching TV
Saturday	12 am	Unknown	8:30 am	Unknown	8:30 am	510/510 × 100 = 100%	Went out with friends
Sunday	10:30 pm	12:30 am	3:00 am	60 min	9:30 am	480/660 × 100 = 73%	
Monday	10:30 pm	11:30 pm	3:00 am	90 min	6:30 am	450/480 × 100 = 94%	Woke up early to take care of grandkids
Tuesday	9:00 pm	10:30 pm	3:00 am	180 min	9:30 am	450/750 × 100 = 60%	

References

1. American Psychiatric Association. Diagnostic and statistical manual of mental disorders. 5th ed., text revised ed. Arlington: Author; 2022.
2. Araújo T, Jarrin DC, Leanza Y, et al. Qualitative studies of insomnia: current state of knowledge in the field. Sleep Med Rev. 2017;31:58–69.
3. Arroll B, Fernando A 3rd, Falloon K, Goodyear-Smith F, Samaranayake C, Warman G. Prevalence of causes of insomnia in primary care: a cross-sectional study. Br J Gen Pract. 2012;62(595):e99–e103. https://doi.org/10.3399/bjgp12X625157.
4. Baranwal N, Yu PK, Siegel NS. Sleep physiology, pathophysiology, and sleep hygiene. Prog Cardiovasc Dis. 2023;77:59–69. https://doi.org/10.1016/j.pcad.2023.02.005.
5. Ben Letaifa S, Charfi F, Ben Hamouda A, Khmekhem R, Hadj Amor S, Fakhfakh R. Validation of Tunisian Arabic version of Pittsburgh Sleep Quality Index in non-clinical adolescents. La Tunisie Medicale. 2024;102(5):278–83. https://doi.org/10.62438/tunismed.v102i5.4929.
6. Buysse DJ, Reynolds CF 3rd, Monk TH, Berman SR, Kupfer DJ. The Pittsburgh Sleep Quality Index: a new instrument for psychiatric practice and research. Psychiatry Res. 1989;28(2):193–213. https://doi.org/10.1016/0165-1781(89)90047-4.
7. Cruz-Sanabria F, Bruno S, Crippa A, Frumento P, Scarselli M, Skene DJ, Faraguna U. Optimizing the time and dose of melatonin as a sleep-promoting drug: A systematic review of randomized controlled trials and dose-response meta-analysis. J Pineal Res. 2024;76(5):e12985. https://doi.org/10.1111/jpi.12985.
8. Desai K, Paladine H, Pilipenko N. Insomnia and sleep disorders in older women. In: Brown HW, Williams M, Schrager S, editors. Challenges in older women's health: a guide for clinicians; 2021. p. 105–23.
9. Ell J, Schmid SR, Benz F, Spille L. Complementary and alternative treatments for insomnia disorder: a systematic umbrella review. J Sleep Res. 2023;32(6):e13979. https://doi.org/10.1111/jsr.13979.
10. Fernandez-Mendoza J, Rodriguez-Muñoz A, Vela-Bueno A, Olavarrieta-Bernardino S, Calhoun SL, Bixler EO, Vgontzas AN. The Spanish version of the Insomnia Severity Index: a confirmatory factor analysis. Sleep Med. 2012;13(2):207–10. https://doi.org/10.1016/j.sleep.2011.06.019.
11. Ferracioli-Oda E, Qawasmi A, Bloch MH. Meta-analysis: melatonin for the treatment of primary sleep disorders. PLoS One. 2013;8(5):e63773. https://doi.org/10.1371/journal.pone.0063773.
12. Gómez-Benito J, Ruiz C, Guilera G. A Spanish version of the Athens Insomnia Scale. Qual Life Res Int J Qual Life Asp Treat Care Rehab. 2011;20(6):931–7. https://doi.org/10.1007/s11136-010-9827-x.
13. Hallit S, Haddad C, Hallit R, Al Karaki G, Malaeb D, Sacre H, Kheir N, Hajj A, Salameh P. Validation of selected sleeping disorders related scales in Arabic among the Lebanese Population. Sleep Biol Rhythms. 2019;17:183–9. https://doi.org/10.1007/s41105-018-0196-0.
14. Hennemann S, Böhme K, Kleinstäuber M, et al. Internet-based CBT for somatic symptom distress (iSOMA) in emerging adults: a randomized controlled trial. J Consult Clin Psychol. 2022;90(4):353–65. https://doi.org/10.1037/ccp0000707.
15. Hita-Contreras F, Martínez-López E, Latorre-Román PA, Garrido F, Santos MA, Martínez-Amat A. Reliability and validity of the Spanish version of the Pittsburgh Sleep Quality Index (PSQI) in patients with fibromyalgia. Rheumatol Int. 2014;34(7):929–36. https://doi.org/10.1007/s00296-014-2960-z.
16. Ji X, Grandner MA, Liu J. The relationship between micronutrient status and sleep patterns: a systematic review. Public Health Nutr. 2017;20(4):687–701. https://doi.org/10.1017/S1368980016002603.
17. Kaufmann CN, Mojtabai R, Hock RS, Thorpe RJ Jr, Canham SL, Chen LY, Wennberg AM, Chen-Edinboro LP, Spira AP. Racial/ethnic differences in insomnia trajectories among

U.S. Older Adults. Am J Geriatr Psychiatry. 2016;24(7):575–84. https://doi.org/10.1016/j.jagp.2016.02.049.
18. Leung W, Singh I, McWilliams S, Stockler S, Ipsiroglu OS. Iron deficiency and sleep – a scoping review. Sleep Med Rev. 2020;51:101274. https://doi.org/10.1016/j.smrv.2020.101274.
19. Matheson EM, Brown BD, Decastro AO. Treatment of chronic insomnia in adults. Am Fam Physician. 2024;109(2):154–60.
20. Morin CM, Belleville G, Bélanger L, Ivers H. The Insomnia Severity Index: psychometric indicators to detect insomnia cases and evaluate treatment response. Sleep. 2011;34(5):601–8. https://doi.org/10.1093/sleep/34.5.601.
21. National Sleep Foundation. How many hours of sleep do you really need? 2020. https://www.thensf.org/how-many-hours-of-sleep-do-you-really-need/
22. Qaseem A, Kansagara D, Forciea MA, Cooke M, Denberg TD, for the Clinical Guidelines Committee of the American College of Physicians. Management of chronic insomnia disorder in adults: A clinical practice guideline from the American College of Physicians. Ann Intern Med. 2016;165(2):125–33. https://doi.org/10.7326/M15-2175.
23. Qaseem A, Kansagara D, Forciea MA, Cooke M, Denberg TD. Clinical guidelines committee of the American College of Physicians. Management of chronic insomnia disorder in adults: a clinical practice guideline from the American College of Physicians. Ann Intern Med. 2016;165(2):125–33. https://doi.org/10.7326/M15-2175.
24. Sateia MJ, Buysse DJ, Krystal AD, Neubauer DN, Heald JL. Clinical practice guideline for the pharmacologic treatment of chronic insomnia in adults: an American Academy of Sleep Medicine clinical practice guideline. J Clin Sleep Med. 2017;13(2):307–49. https://doi.org/10.5664/jcsm.6470.
25. Shaha DP. Insomnia management: a review and update. J Fam Pract. 2023;72(6 Suppl):S31–6. https://doi.org/10.12788/jfp.0620.
26. Shapour BA, Gang CK. Reliability and validity of the Chinese translation of Insomnia Severity Index and comparison with Pittsburgh Sleep Quality Index. Malays J Psychiatry. 2013;22(2):3–9. https://doi.org/10.1016/S0924-9338(13)77338-3.
27. Soldatos CR, Dikeos DG, Paparrigopoulos TJ. Athens insomnia scale: validation of an instrument based on ICD-10 criteria. J Psychosom Res. 2000;48(6):555–60. https://doi.org/10.1016/s0022-3999(00)00095-7.
28. Soldatos CR, Dikeos DG, Paparrigopoulos TJ. The diagnostic validity of the Athens Insomnia Scale. J Psychosom Res. 2003;55(3):263–7. https://doi.org/10.1016/s0022-3999(02)00604-9.
29. Suleiman KH, Yates BC. Translating the insomnia severity index into Arabic. J Nurs Sch. 2011;43(1):49–53. https://doi.org/10.1111/j.1547-5069.2010.01374.x.
30. Sutton EL. Insomnia. Ann Intern Med. 2021;174(3):ITC33–48. https://doi.org/10.7326/AITC202103160.
31. Tan C, Wang J, Cao G, Chen C, Yin J, Lu J, Qiu J. Reliability and validity of the Chinese version of the Athens insomnia scale for non-clinical application in Chinese athletes. Front Psychol. 2023;14:1183919. https://doi.org/10.3389/fpsyg.2023.11839.
32. van Straten A, van der Zweerde T, Kleiboer A, Cuijpers P, Morin CM, Lancee J. Cognitive and behavioral therapies in the treatment of insomnia: a meta-analysis. Sleep Med Rev. 2018;38:3–16. https://doi.org/10.1016/j.smrv.2017.02.001.
33. Winkelman JW. Insomnia disorder. N Engl J Med. 2015;373:1437–44.
34. Wong VW, Ho FY, Wong YS, Chung KF, Yeung WF, Ng CH, Sarris J. Efficacy of lifestyle medicine on sleep quality: a meta-analysis of randomized controlled trials. J Affect Disord. 2023;330:125–38. https://doi.org/10.1016/j.jad.2023.02.111.
35. Zhang C, Zhang H, Zhao M, Li Z, Cook CE, Buysse DJ, Zhao Y, Yao Y. Reliability, validity, and factor structure of Pittsburgh sleep quality index in community-based centenarians. Front Psych. 2020;11:573530. https://doi.org/10.3389/fpsyt.2020.573530.
36. Zhao M, Tuo H, Wang S, Zhao L. The effects of dietary nutrition on sleep and sleep disorders. Mediators Inflamm. 2020;2020:3142874. https://doi.org/10.1155/2020/3142874.

Part II
Pain-Related Conditions

Chapter 6
Chronic Pain

Kimberly A. Muellers, Stella D. Nelms, and Krishna M. Desai

Case Vignette

Mrs. F is a 35-year-old woman presenting for follow-up of chronic, progressive pain involving the back, neck, bilateral hands, knees, and abdomen. Imaging studies revealed mild degenerative changes in the spine, normal radiographs of both hands, and normal abdominal and pelvic computed tomography scans with no evidence of intra-abdominal pathology.

Mrs. F: *I'm fed up! I've tried everything and I'm still in pain every day!*

Dr. D: *I'm sorry to hear you're feeling frustrated. What strategies have you tried since our last visit?*

Mrs. F: *Well I tried the gabapentin you gave me last time, which helps some. When I don't take gabapentin I use Tylenol, but it only helps a little. I use lidocaine patches every day but I'm still in pain.*

K. A. Muellers (✉)
Department of Psychology, The New School for Social Research, New York, NY, USA

Department of Psychology, Pace University, New York, NY, USA
e-mail: kmuellers@pace.edu

S. D. Nelms
Division of Neuropsychology and Behavioral Health, Department of Rehabilitation Medicine, Emory University School of Medicine, Atlanta, GA, USA

K. M. Desai
Center for Family and Community Medicine, Department of Medicine, Columbia University Irving Medical Center/New York Presbyterian Hospital, New York, NY, USA

Center for Neuroinflammatory and Somatic Disorders, Department of Psychiatry, Columbia University Irving Medical Center/New York Presbyterian Hospital, New York, NY, USA

N. Pilipenko, K. M. Desai (eds.), *8 Conditions Primary Care Clinicians Dread to Treat*, https://doi.org/10.1007/978-3-032-12819-5_6

Dr. D: *I see, so medications help some but they don't fully resolve your pain. Besides medications, what else have you tried?*

Mrs. F: *When the pain is too bad I usually lie down and maybe take a nap. I'm not sure what else I could be doing.*

Dr. D: *I see. And how would you rate your pain before and after taking medication, on a scale from 0 to 10?*

Mrs. F: *Before medication I would say 8/10; after I take gabapentin and use the patch it's maybe 6/10. But I just want it to stop. Some days I don't think I can take this pain any longer!*

Dr. D: *Sounds like you have been really suffering. What do you expect will happen with your pain over time?*

Mrs. F: *I don't know, I'm hoping it will go away but the longer this goes on, the less I believe it will.*

Dr. D: *Your pain has been going on for a long time now: because it has lasted more than three months, we consider this to be* ***chronic pain (CP)****. What does the diagnosis mean to you?*

Mrs. F: *I'm not sure. I thought maybe spine damage caused my back and neck pain, but you said everything looks fine. I don't know why my hands and knees hurt. Maybe we haven't found the right medication.*

Dr. D: *What do you hope would happen if we found the right medication?*

Mrs. F: *Ideally, the pain would go away!*

Dr. D: [Messages #1 and #2].

Dr. D provides resources (see Education for Patients) and asks Mrs. F to view the videos before her next follow-up.

Diagnosis: Brief Description

CP is defined as pain that "persists or recurs for more than three months" [54, p. 19]. According to the International Classification of Diseases, **CP** is "primary" if it is not caused by another known condition. Alternatively **CP** can be described by a secondary pain disorder: cancer-related, neuropathic, visceral, posttraumatic/surgical, headache/orofacial, or musculoskeletal pain [54]. Patients with **CP** may also meet criteria for Somatic Symptom Disorder with Pain specifier if pain is accompanied by: 1. Excessive/recurring thoughts about seriousness of pain, 2. High pain-related anxiety, and/or 3. Excessive pain focus [3]. See Chap. 2 for further discussion.

CP is frequently underdiagnosed in primary care (PC), leading to excess healthcare costs and reduced treatment effectiveness [5]. When poorly managed, **CP** is linked to significant distress, poor quality of life, functional impairment, and low treatment satisfaction [28]. Unlike acute pain, **CP** does not typically arise from a single causal event. Rather, it occurs through a combination of biological, psychological, and social factors [19]. **CP** is heterogeneous and likely encompasses multiple etiologies [48].

Prevalence, Risk Factors, and Disparities

In the U.S., **CP** affects 20% of the general population [6] and 33% of PC patients [5]. Risk factors include older age, female sex, racial/ethnic minority status, lower socioeconomic status, limited education, unemployment, and low occupational autonomy [28]. Lifestyle factors such as smoking, alcohol use, physical inactivity, low vitamin D, and diet further elevate **CP** risk [19].

Clinical risk factors include diagnosed pain-related conditions, chronic illness, history of postoperative pain, obesity, and insomnia [28]. History of injury, abuse, or trauma also predict greater **CP** risk [19].

Bias and stereotyping contribute to underdiagnosis and undertreatment of **CP** among Black, Indigenous, and People of Color (BIPOC). Clinical judgment may be skewed by two seemingly contrasting myths: that BIPOC patients have higher pain tolerance, or that they tend to overreport pain. Thus, BIPOC patients receive less aggressive **CP** treatment compared to non-Hispanic White patients [31]. Restricted access to **CP** treatment combined with long-term effects of discrimination on stress regulation may explain why BIPOC patients report more severe, persistent **CP** and greater negative impacts on quality of life [35, 55]. Furthermore, **CP** in patients with a history of illicit substance use may be dismissed due to suspicions of drug-seeking behavior [44].

Symptom Assessment Tools

Patient-reported outcome measures are essential to **CP** diagnosis and management. The 0–10 pain rating scale frequently utilized in PC demonstrates "only modest accuracy for identifying patients with clinically important pain" [22]. Several more effective tools for **CP** assessment are available (Table 6.1). The Brief Pain Inventory (BPI, [52]) assesses overall pain-related severity and interference. If neuropathic pain is suspected, the ID Pain measure [38] may be appropriate. The Pain Catastrophizing Scale [50] helps to identify patients at risk for greater pain intensity, emotional distress, and functional impairment.

In clinical interviews, the "ACT-UP" approach can be used. This involves asking patients about: pain's impact on *A*ctivities, *C*oping, *T*houghts about pain, being *U*pset about pain, and other *P*eople's responses towards pain [7].

Table 6.1 Chronic pain screening tools

Screener Name	Items #	Rating scale scoring	Cut offs	Assessment timeline	Availability	Psychometric properties	Non-English Versions Available?
Brief pain inventory-short form (BPI)	9 [52]	11-point rating scale [52] 0 = no pain to 10 = pain as bad as you can imagine	No cutoffs; use "worst" rating or mean of 4 ratings to determine pain severity [25, 52]	Past 24 h [52]	Open access [52]	Internal consistency:.85 [52] Test-retest reliability:.70 [20] to.85 [27] Appropriate convergent and discriminant validity [46] Sensitivity: 79.37%, specificity: 46.9%, positive predictive value: 65.8% compared to clinical assessment [10]	Arabic, Chinese, Spanish [25]
ID pain	6 [38]	Yes/No items (5 items scored +1 for yes, 1 item −1 for no) [38]	Likelihood of neuropathic pain: [15] 4–5 likely 2–3 probable 0 or − 1 improbable	Current pain [38]	Open access	Good convergent validity with other neuropathic pain scales [36] Good discriminant validity to detect neuropathic vs. nociceptive pain; sensitivity 78% and specificity 74% [36] Predictive validity 0.72 compared to clinician diagnosis [40]	Arabic [1], Chinese [56], Spanish [12]
Pain catastrophizing scale (PCS)	13 [50]	5-point Likert scale [50] 0 = Not at all to 4 = All the time	Cut offs 30 indicates clinically relevant levels [50] Sub-scores for rumination, magnification, and helplessness [12]	No timeline	Open access [24]	Internal consistency = 0.92–0.95 in community and outpatient samples [34] Significant correlation with depression and anxiety, more strongly correlated with pain than mood [30]	Arabic [18], Chinese [57], Spanish [13]

Non-pharmacological Conceptualization: What to Say to the Patient?

Effective **CP** management requires a biopsychosocial approach that integrates biological, psychological, and social factors alongside pharmacological treatments [17]. Despite growing recognition of the biopsychosocial model's importance in **CP** care, practical guidance for integrating non-pharmacological interventions remains limited. The following section outlines key messages for patients regarding non-pharmacological **CP** management.

Message #1: Chronic Pain Is Different from Acute Pain

When an acute injury occurs, pain is regulated by brain-body mechanisms. For example, if your hand touches a flame, the body automatically withdraws the hand to prevent further harm. Although this response is coordinated by the brain, it happens almost instantly and without conscious thought. In cases of acute pain, the primary goal is to protect the body and allow healing. Typically, healing is completed within approximately 3 months.

In **CP**, however, pain signals continue after tissue healing is complete. This happens because the nervous system becomes more sensitive. Imagine your body contains "gates" that prevent pain from traveling from your foot to your brain, for example. Normally, the gate stays closed and you feel no pain. In **CP**, the body's ability to keep the gate closed gets weaker, meaning the gate opens even when you aren't injured, causing pain. This change happens due to factors like negative emotions, inactivity, stress, and a sense of loss of control, all of which can amplify the pain experience. Even safe signals, such as light touch or normal movement, may be interpreted as threatening [32].

This means that the brain and nervous system (the home of the "gates") play a key role in **CP**. This does not make the pain any less real, but it does mean that **CP** requires different solutions than acute pain.

Why? Educating patients about the difference between acute and **CP** via the gate-control theory of pain is essential for improving outcomes. Evidence for the gate-control theory suggests that experiences of **CP** relate to changes in the balance of input from large-nerve fibers, which "shut the gate" or inhibit pain signals, and small-nerve fibers, which "open the gate" allowing pain signals to travel to the brain [26]. Over time, the number of large-nerve fibers connected to the pain site decreases, making the "gate" more prone to opening in response to physiological and psychological inputs. When physicians explain that **CP** does not necessarily mean ongoing tissue damage, patients are more likely to reengage in physical activity, reduce catastrophizing, and perceive **CP** as less disabling [23, 32].

Message #2: CP Treatment Aims to Reduce Pain, Not to Cure It

Most people wish to get rid of **CP** completely. This wish is very understandable. Unfortunately, for **CP** treatment total pain elimination is not always possible. Typically, reduction of pain by half is considered a success. The main focus of **CP** care is improving functioning: being able to do meaningful and important activities with minimum limitations.

Why? Complete **CP** elimination is rare; a 30–50% pain reduction is considered to be a clinically meaningful outcome [41]. However, many patients focus on pain elimination as their primary goal, leading to a cycle of cure-seeking and increased frustration which can negatively affect **CP** control. Clear communication about realistic goals improves treatment satisfaction [29].

Message #3: CP Management Requires a Range of Interventions

The way your body experiences **CP** is affected by many factors. Therefore multiple strategies are needed to improve **CP**, including changes to physical activity, stress management, and thoughts and emotions related to pain. You can use a combination of techniques to reduce daily pain and improve quality of life. This includes changing how you think about pain (Technique #1), **pacing** your activities to prevent pain from getting worse (Technique #2), and gradually increasing your physical abilities and improving mood through enjoyable activities (Technique #3).

See Resources section for patient-friendly videos explaining these concepts.

Why? The emotional impacts of **CP** have important implications for treatment outcomes [17], and thus addressing psychological and lifestyle factors can decrease pain intensity and interference in daily life [42]. It is important for patients to understand that **CP** treatment will involve multiple approaches, and that these techniques require daily engagement and produce gradual progress.

When available, physicians can consider working with an interdisciplinary team to support care delivery [43]. Involvement of interdisciplinary team members (mental/behavioral health providers, physical, occupational, and recreational therapists) offers patients access to evidence-based techniques and tools beyond the PCP's scope of practice.

Case Vignette—Continued

Mrs. F returns for follow-up 4 weeks later. Dr. D stops to greet her in the waiting area and asks if she was able to review **CP** materials. Mrs. F says she "forgot." Dr. D helps her locate the "5-Minute Pain video" (See Resources) and asks her to review it while she waits for her visit.

The following discussion takes place during the visit.

Dr. D: *What did you think about the video?*

Mrs. F: *It was okay. It said my pain may never go away completely—is that true?*

Dr. D: *If complete relief isn't possible, what pain level would let you enjoy life and do the things you want?*

Mrs. F: *Maybe 4/10?*

Dr. D: *Ok, so at 4 you could live your life even though the pain would still be there. Based on what we know about* ***CP****, I would like to focus on reaching a 4 instead of a 0 as a realistic goal. [Uses Message #1 to educate].*

Through further conversation, Dr. D learns that Mrs. F uses gabapentin inconsistently and tends to wait until pain peaks before taking Tylenol.

Dr. D: *It sounds like you took gabapentin 3 times last week and used Tylenol 6 out of 7 days. What usually happens that leads you to take Tylenol?*

Mrs. F: *I take it when the pain becomes too much. On Sunday it was when my hands and knees got so bad I had to stop doing laundry and go lie down.*

Dr. D: *So you're taking Tylenol only when the pain is severe. Have any of your providers discussed with you when it's best to take Tylenol?*

Mrs. F: *No.*

Dr. D: *Can I tell you about what is currently recommended for taking pain medication in* ***CP****?*

Mrs. F: *Sure.*

Dr. D: *This may seem surprising, but we find that pain medications are more effective if you take them before the pain is at its worst. What do you think about this idea?*

What concerns do you have about taking gabapentin daily?

Mrs. F: *Well on days where I feel ok, I don't want to take medication. I'm worried that if I take it too much, I'll be dependent on it.*

Dr. D: *That's understandable. Luckily, gabapentin does not cause dependency, and it actually works better if you take it every day, even when your pain is lower. How does it sound if we set a goal for you to try taking gabapentin every day until our next appointment and see how that affects your pain levels?*

Mrs. F: *Ok.*

Non-pharmacological Treatment Options: What Can Be Done?

1. **Address Catastrophic CP Beliefs**

   Patients' appraisal of **CP** affects both emotion and behaviors, including illness management. **CP**-related thoughts are important predictors of treatment success [48], and patients with **CP** frequently experience *catastrophizing*. Pain catastrophizing has been conceptualized as a combination of three unhelpful patterns of appraisal: magnification ("My pain keeps getting worse!"), rumination ("I can't stop thinking about the pain"), and helplessness ("There is nothing I can do to make the pain go away") [50]. Catastrophizing may result from attentional bias toward pain-related stimuli, seeking interpersonal support, and/or changes to neural mechanisms involved in pain response [39]. Although some patients and researchers critique the term "catastrophizing" as dismissive and potentially stigmatizing, other experts argue this connotation arises because providers fail to apply the biopsychosocial model (i.e. discounting biological factors because psychological factors are present; [51]). Effective **CP** care should involve assessment for pain catastrophizing, and if present, addressing its role in **CP** maintenance in conjunction with other techniques.

How to address? Cognitive disputation (CD) helps patients replace unhelpful beliefs about **CP** with balanced thoughts [17]. See Chap. 2 for a detailed description. In the context of **CP**, even a single **CD** session can improve pain-related outcomes. One trial demonstrated large reductions in pain catastrophizing following a two-hour intervention including psychoeducation and training in **CD** and relaxation ($d = 0.85$ at 2 weeks and $d = 1.15$ at 4 weeks; [8]).

2. **Teach Skills to Manage Cycles of Over/Under-activity**

   Patients with **CP** often either "push through" pain or overexert themselves on "good days" resulting in subsequent pain exacerbations. Over/under activity leads pain to become associated with physical activity, while rest becomes associated with pain reduction. The result is that exertion becomes negatively reinforced: cessation or decrease of pain becomes associated with inactivity, which in turn strengthens this behavior as a coping mechanism. However, this cycle causes poorer physical and psychological functioning [4].

   How to address? Activity **pacing** teaches the patient to engage in timed periods of activity and rest, avoiding pain exacerbations [14]. Prior to beginning activity **pacing** intervention, physicians should ensure that the patient understands how **CP** operates (see Message #1).

   Pacing involves the following steps:

   1. Help the patient identify an activity they can do every day. Instruct the patient to begin the activity and check in with themselves every few minutes to assess pain and fatigue. Once fatigue increases, they should stop the activity, note how long they engaged, then rest and record how long it takes to recover. This will provide data for setting appropriate periods of time to engage in activity and rest without exacerbating pain or causing fatigue.

      (a) For example, Mrs. F states that she needs to wash her dishes but becomes fatigued by the time she completes the task. After reviewing with Dr. D, she discovers that she can wash dishes for 15 min before becoming fatigued, and she needs to sit for 10 min before feeling ready to resume activity.

   2. The patient should develop a plan to engage in the activity for a set length of time, followed by a set period of rest, prior to re-engaging in activity. This strategy decouples experiences of activity and pain by preventing pain exacerbations.

(a) Mrs. F and Dr. D plan that Mrs. F will wash dishes daily after dinner for 15 min or until she feels fatigued, then rest on the couch and listen to music for 10 min before returning to the dishes. She will repeat this cycle until the task is complete.

3. Instruct the patient to track progress and commit to a structured **pacing** schedule for 1–2 weeks before adjusting the lengths of activity and rest periods if needed. The patient can gradually increase activity as long as pain "spikes" are avoided [19].

   (a) Mrs. F uses a timer to track her activity and rest periods and a symptom tracking app (see Resources) to monitor her pain and fatigue levels before and after washing dishes each day.

3. **Focus on Increasing Activities**

CP frequently leads to withdrawal from social and physical activities due to fear of pain exacerbation [4]. Activity avoidance in **CP** is associated with reduced physical and occupational functioning and increased depressive symptoms [16].

How to address? Behavioral activation (BA) involves increasing activities that are enjoyable or rewarding, decreasing avoidance, and helping patients problem-solve barriers to these goals. **BA** techniques are both feasible and acceptable in PC [49].

The following steps are involved (adapted from [49]):

1. Patient education: Explain that many patients with **CP** limit or avoid activities because they fear worsening pain. Discuss specific examples of avoidance in the patient's daily life. Ask about enjoyable or meaningful activities that the patient has reduced or stopped because of **CP** and identify activities they would like to resume.

   (a) Mrs. F says she used to enjoy evening walks with her friend but has stopped since her **CP** worsened.

2. Activity tracking: Ask the patient to track weekly activity and note corresponding pain and mood levels. Review tracking logs together to identify activities that are enjoyable and rewarding and those used as avoidance.

   (a) Mrs. F notes enjoying dinner with her sister and feeling accomplished for attending despite anxiety about pain. She identified lying on the couch and looking at social media as an avoidance behavior.

3. Goal Setting: Help the patient select an enjoyable, rewarding activity and develop a realistic, detailed plan for doing it. Establish *S*pecific, *M*easurable, *A*chievable, *R*elevant, and *T*ime-bound (SMART) behavioral goals (see Resources). Set one goal at a time. Instruct the patient to engage in the scheduled behavior even if they are "not in the mood."

   (a) Dr. D and Mrs. F decide she will walk with her friend in the park at 6 pm three times per week for 20 min each time. She will try this weekly until her next appointment and track activity completion, mood, and pain levels.

4. Follow-up and problem solving: Review the patient's progress at follow-up visits. If the patient has difficulty completing the goal, help them problem-solve: identify barriers, brainstorm, and select a strategy to overcome them.
   (a) Mrs. F's friend is only available two nights per week. She arranges to walk with another friend on Saturday mornings.

Psychotherapy Effectiveness

Psychotherapy can help patients learn effective strategies for coping with **CP**. Cognitive behavioral therapy for **CP** (CBT-CP) demonstrates small effects in reducing pain intensity ($d = -0.18$), pain interference ($d = -0.13$), catastrophizing (d = −0.18), depression (d = −0.13), and anxiety (d = −0.21) across patient populations with varying pain sites and **CP** etiologies. These results correspond to a decrease in pain intensity of 0.49 on a 0–10 scale and a decrease in catastrophizing of 0.32 on a 0–6 scale [33].

Evidence on the duration of CBT-CP benefits is mixed. A meta-analysis found that reductions in pain intensity ($d = -0.25$), but not other outcomes, persisted at 6 months posttreatment [33]. One study demonstrated moderate-to-large and long-lasting effects including reduced pain intensity (1 year: $d = 0.46$, 3 years: $d = 0.33$), pain interference (1 year: $d = 0.59$, 3 years: $d = 0.60$), depression (1 year: $d = 0.46$; 3 years: $d = 0.39$), and psychological inflexibility (1 year: $d = 0.88$, 3 years: $d = 0.59$; [2]). These findings represent an average change in pain intensity from 7.27 to 6.47 out of 10 at 1-year and 6.50 at 3-year follow-up, and an average reduction in pain interference from 4.69 on a 0–6 scale to 4.07 at 1-year and 3.89 at 3-year follow-up [2].

Group psychotherapy may be more effective than individual sessions in reducing pain intensity (group: $d = -0.20$, individual: $d = -0.12$; [33]). CBT-CP can be effectively delivered in-person or online [21].

Nonetheless, CBT-CP is not universally effective, reducing pain intensity in 43% of studies [21]. Thus, physicians should set realistic expectations: CBT-CP may improve psychological and physical symptoms related to **CP** for many, but not all, patients.

Integrative Medicine Interventions and Techniques

Relaxation training: Breathing retraining exercises, meditation, and guided imagery are evidence-supported for **CP** and can reduce anxiety, stress, and focus on pain. A daily practice of 5 to 10 min per day can be recommended to patients [48].

Encouraging daily relaxation practice even on "good" days is important for long-term success [17].

Biofeedback: **Biofeedback** involves training patients to monitor and ultimately self-regulate physiological responses in the body [11]. It is effective as a standalone or adjunctive treatment for multiple **CP** conditions. Meta-analysis indicates large effects of **biofeedback** in reducing pain intensity (Hedges' g = 0.60) with outcomes maintained 8 months post-intervention. Additional benefits included small effects of reduced disability (Hedges' $g = 0.49$), reduced muscle tension (Hedges' $g = 0.44$), and improved coping (Hedges' g = 0.41; [45]). Physicians can use the video provided in the Resources section to explain how **biofeedback** works.

Herbs/Botanicals/Supplements (HBS):

St. John's Wort (SJW): A small placebo-controlled RCT evaluated the effectiveness of topical SJW oil on chronic knee osteoarthritis and found a significant difference in mean Visual Analog Score (VAS) after three weeks of treatment. The mean VAS score decreased two-fold in the experimental group compared with the control group ($p < .05$; [47]). Patients can either purchase SJW oil or make their own infusion. Topical SJW can cause photosensitivity so patients should be advise to protect skin from direct sun exposure.

Instructions for making SJW oil (adapted from [47]):

1. Place SJW flowers in a glass jar.
2. Pour enough olive oil to completely cover the flowers.
3. Use a utensil to push down the flowers to ensure they are fully submerged.
4. Set the jar in a warm, sunny spot for 15 days.
5. Strain the oil and apply to clean skin three times per day for three weeks.
6. Avoid sun exposure to the skin where oil is applied to prevent skin irritation from photosensitivity.

Turmeric (curcumin) supplements are effective in reducing **CP** related to osteoarthritis. A systematic review of studies comparing the effect of turmeric with placebo or non-steroidal anti-inflammatory drugs (NSAIDs) on osteoarthritis-related chronic knee pain demonstrated that turmeric reduces pain and improves function similarly to NSAIDs but with fewer adverse effects. Turmeric was also a safe adjunctive treatment, leading to additive pain relief when used with NSAIDs and reduced the dose requirement for NSAIDs. Four studies comparing the effects of turmeric versus placebo on osteoarthritis pain scores demonstrated large effect sizes (0.8–4.1), indicating substantial clinical benefit in pain and function outcomes associated with turmeric supplementation [37]. Turmeric is not readily bioavailable, therefore physicians should recommend products which maximize bioavailability (e.g. micellar formulations; colloidal submicro-particle dispersions; combined with bioperine). Doses of 1000-1500 mg divided into two to three doses per day can be recommended [53].

Capsaicin is the active compound in chili peppers and can be used to treat chronic neuropathic pain. A systematic review demonstrated that at 8 and 12 weeks, about 10% more participants with postherpetic neuralgia reported their pain was "very much improved" with capsaicin cream than with "active" placebo, with numbers needed to treat (NNT) of 8.8 (95% CI: 5.3, 26) with high-concentration capsaicin. Capsaicin is available over the counter in doses ranging from 0.025–0.1%. Patients can expect mild local skin reactions when capsaicin cream is initiated but they usually get better over time with consistent use [9].

Clinical Pearls

- Explain the biopsychosocial model of **CP** to patients early in treatment. Normalize the effects of **CP** on thoughts, emotions, and behaviors, and utilize screening tools that capture these elements of the **CP** experience.
- Use psychoeducation to ensure realistic expectations of **CP** control.
- Provide patients with multiple tools to regulate physical and psychological **CP** symptoms, including **CD**, activity **pacing**, **BA**, relaxation, and HBS.

Frequently Asked Questions

Question 1: *Are you saying I should just 'give up' on solving my pain? What if there's a cure we haven't found yet?*

Answer: Not at all—but a complete cure may not be realistic. I am recommending that we work together to help you develop pain coping techniques. These could help you feel better and make it more possible to do the things that are important to you in spite of your pain.

Question 2: *I'm not sure if BA will work for me. I want to start walking again, but my pain is so bad sometimes I don't see how I can do anything without making it worse!*

Answer: It can be scary to become more active. This is why we'll start small to prevent the pain from getting worse. We can treat this as an experiment to see how walking affects your mood and your pain.

Question 3: *Why should I see a psychologist for pain? I don't see how they'll help.*

Answer: It may be surprising, but cognitive behavioral therapy uses the science of **CP** to teach strategies that can change how you think, feel, and act toward your pain. With this treatment, some patients feel less overwhelmed or depressed and experience less pain. CBT-CP can reduce pain by about 0.5 on a 0–10 scale, and can reduce catastrophic thinking about **CP** by about 6%. Thus, it can be one source of potential improvement when used alongside other coping skills.

Case Vignette: Conclusion

Dr. D and Mrs. F met three months later to discuss her **CP** treatment plan, address concerns, and review the conceptualization.

Dr. D: *What questions do you have for me after watching the videos?*

Mrs. F: *I guess I'm wondering if it's really possible to reduce my pain by doing more activities. I hadn't thought about it before, but when the pain is bad I usually avoid going out. But if I need to run a small errand, I feel a bit better afterward.*

Dr. D: *I'm glad you've noticed this pattern. What you're describing fits our understanding of* ***pacing*** *and how the right balance of activity and rest can help minimize pain. How do you think you could use this approach in your day-to-day life?*

Mrs. F: *I could try doing small errands every day instead of waiting to do everything on a day when my pain is low?*

Dr. D: *Right. And I also want to talk about how you can take your pain medications in a way that will give them the best chance of helping you. Is it okay if we spend the next few minutes making a plan for these two strategies together?*

Mrs. F: *Ok.*

Mrs. F agreed to practice activity **pacing**, try using medications before pain reaches its peak, and monitor her daily pain levels. Dr. D asked the clinic's social worker to connect Mrs. F with an online **CP** support group. Mrs. F will return in three months to review progress.

Resources

Source	Description	Link
Education for Patients		
"Understanding Pain in Less than Five Minutes"	Animated video explaining CP Duration: 5:00	https://youtu.be/5KrUL8tOaQs?si=zPqJRNyY2fXXhcjJ
"Understanding Pain: Brainman Chooses"	Animated video explaining role of the brain in CP Duration: 2:29	https://youtu.be/jIwn9rC3rOI?si=NeSLdUj8cQ76Fkfc
"Tame the Beast: It's Time to Rethink Persistent Pain"	Animated overview of CP mechanisms and how to reduce CP symptoms Duration: 5:00	https://youtu.be/ikUzvSph7Z4?si=voi9WiekqesgvCt5
Why things hurt	TED Talk on CP Duration: 14:32	https://www.youtube.com/watch?v=gwd-wLdIHjs
Introduction to Biofeedback	Patient-friendly explanation of biofeedback Duration: 5:09	https://www.youtube.com/watch?v=BP4MYftF9Ao
Phone apps (Tracking, relaxation)		
Branch	Free app with symptom tracking and social aspects	https://appadvice.com/app/branch-health/1065632442
UT Physicians	Guided meditation for pain Duration: 4:37	https://www.youtube.com/watch?v=T_5S_DhnujY
Insight timer	Free app with relaxation exercises	https://insighttimer.com/

(continued)

Source	Description	Link
UCLA Mindful	Free app with meditations	https://www.uclahealth.org/ulcamindful/ucla-mindful-app
Smiling Mind	Free app with mood and symptom tracking, relaxation	https://www.smilingmind.com.au/smiling-mind-app
Instructions/Guides for Providers		
Brief Behavioral Skills: Behavioral Activation	Video guide for providers on BA Duration: 37:52	https://youtu.be/fqk41YZ81uM?si=r9_tvqYSccv1JEEh
SMART Goals Guide	Fillable PDF guide to set SMART goals with patients	https://www.acpe-accredit.org/pdf/CPD/CAP_SMART_Goal_Guide.pdf
U.S. Veterans Association	Provider guide to acupressure for low back pain	https://news.va.gov/102726/live-whole-health-120-acupressure-puts-low-back-pain-relief-in-your-fingertips/ https://www.va.gov/files/2021-12/4309_Acupressure_For_Back_Pain.pdf
U.S. Veterans Association	Provider guide to acupressure for headaches	https://news.va.gov/88566/live-whole-health-72-managing-headaches-acupressure/
U.S. Veterans Association	Overview and video resources on CBT-CP	https://www.va.gov/PAINMANAGEMENT/CBT_CP/Providers.asp
AAFP	Tips for behavioral health management in PC	https://www.aafp.org/pubs/fpm/issues/2017/0300/p30.html
Digital Therapeutics		
Kaia Health	Digital therapeutic app with evidence for musculoskeletal CP	https://kaiahealth.com/
Biofeedback	Video explaining biofeedback technique	https://www.youtube.com/watch?v=BP4MYftF9Ao

References

1. Abu-Shaheen A, Yousef S, Riaz M, Nofal A, Khan S, Heena H. Validity and reliability of Arabic version of the ID Pain screening questionnaire in the assessment of neuropathic pain. PLoS One. 2018;13(3):e0192307. https://doi.org/10.1371/journal.pone.0192307.
2. Åkerblom S, McCracken LM, Rivano Fischer M, Perrin S. Long-term pain and health economic outcomes in adults receiving multidisciplinary CBT for chronic pain: the role of psychological inflexibility. Front Pain Res (Lausanne). 2025;6:1547540. https://doi.org/10.3389/fpain.2025.1547540.
3. American Psychiatric Association. Diagnostic and statistical manual of mental disorders. 5th ed., text rev ed. American Psychiatric Association; 2022. https://doi.org/10.1176/appi.books.9780890425787.
4. Andrews NE, Strong J, Meredith PJ. The relationship between approach to activity engagement, specific aspects of physical function, and pain duration in chronic pain. Clin J Pain. 2016;32(1):20–31. https://doi.org/10.1097/AJP.0000000000000226.

5. Bifulco L, Anderson DR, Blankson ML, Channamsetty V, Blaz JW, Nguyen-Louie TT, Scholle SH. Evaluation of a chronic pain screening program implemented in primary care. JAMA Netw Open. 2021;4(7):e2118495. https://doi.org/10.1001/jamanetworkopen.2021.18495.
6. Dahlhamer J, Lucas J, Zelaya C, Nahin R, Mackey S, DeBar L, Kerns R, Von Korff M, Porter L, Helmick C. Prevalence of chronic pain and high-impact chronic pain among adults—United States, 2016. MMWR Morb Mortal Wkly Rep. 2018;67(36):1001–6. https://doi.org/10.15585/mmwr.mm6736a2.
7. Dansie EJ, Turk DC. Assessment of patients with chronic pain. Br J Anaesth. 2013;111(1):19–25. https://doi.org/10.1093/bja/aet124.
8. Darnall BD, Sturgeon JA, Kao M-C, Hah JM, Mackey SC. From catastrophizing to recovery: a pilot study of a single-session treatment for pain catastrophizing. J Pain Res. 2014;7:219–26. https://doi.org/10.2147/JPR.S62329.
9. Derry S, Rice AS, Cole P, Tan T, Moore RA. Topical capsaicin (high concentration) for chronic neuropathic pain in adults. Cochrane Database Syst Rev. 2017;1(1):CD007393. https://doi.org/10.1002/14651858.CD007393.pub4.
10. Erdemoglu ÂK, Koc R. Brief Pain Inventory score identifying and discriminating neuropathic and nociceptive pain. Acta Neurol Scand. 2013;128(5):351–8. https://doi.org/10.1111/ane.12131.
11. Frank DL, Khorshid L, Kiffer JF, Moravec CS, McKee MG. Biofeedback in medicine: who, when, why and how? Ment Health Fam Med. 2010;7(2):85–91.
12. Gálvez R, Pardo A, Cerón JM, Villasante F, Aranguren JL, Saldaña MT, Navarro A, Ruiz MA, Díaz S, Rejas J. Linguistic adaptation into Spanish and psychometric validation of the ID-Pain questionnaire for the screening of neuropathic pain. Med Clin. 2008;131(15):572–8. https://doi.org/10.1157/13128018.
13. García Campayo J, Rodero B, Alda M, Sobradiel N, Montero J, Moreno S. Validation of the Spanish version of the pain catastrophizing scale in fibromyalgia. Med Clin. 2008;131(13):487–92. https://doi.org/10.1157/13127277.
14. Guy L, McKinstry C, Bruce C. Effectiveness of pacing as a learned strategy for people with chronic pain: a systematic review. Am J Occup Ther. 2019;73(3):7303205060p1-7303205060p10. https://doi.org/10.5014/ajot.2019.028555.
15. Haanpää M, Attal N, Backonja M, Baron R, Bennett M, Bouhassira D, Cruccu G, Hansson P, Haythornthwaite JA, Iannetti GD, Jensen TS, Kauppila T, Nurmikko TJ, Rice ASC, Rowbotham M, Serra J, Sommer C, Smith BH, Treede R-D. NeuPSIG guidelines on neuropathic pain assessment. Pain. 2011;152(1):14–27. https://doi.org/10.1016/j.pain.2010.07.031.
16. Hooker SA, Slattengren AH, Boyle L, Sherman MD. Values-based behavioral activation for chronic pain in primary care: a pilot study. J Clin Psychol Med Settings. 2020;27(4):633–42. https://doi.org/10.1007/s10880-019-09655-x.
17. Hosey M, McWhorter JW, Wegener ST. Psychologic interventions for chronic pain. In: Benzon HT, Raja SN, Liu SS, Fishman SM, Cohen SP, editors. Essentials of pain medicine. 4th ed. Elsevier; 2018. p. 539–544.e1. https://doi.org/10.1016/B978-0-323-40196-8.00059-0.
18. Huijer HA-S, Fares S, French DJ. The development and psychometric validation of an Arabic-language version of the pain catastrophizing scale. Pain Res Manag. 2017:1472792. https://doi.org/10.1155/2017/1472792.
19. Hunter CL, Goodie JL, Oordt MS, Dobmeyer AC. Pain disorders. In: Integrated behavioral health in primary care. 2nd ed. American Psychological Association; 2022. p. 231–56.
20. Keller S, Bann CM, Dodd SL, Schein J, Mendoza TR, Cleeland CS. Validity of the brief pain inventory for use in documenting the outcomes of patients with noncancer pain. Clin J Pain. 2004;20(5):309–18. https://doi.org/10.1097/00002508-200409000-00005.
21. Knoerl R, Lavoie Smith EM, Weisberg J. Chronic pain and cognitive behavioral therapy: an integrative review. West J Nurs Res. 2016;38(5):596–628. https://doi.org/10.1177/0193945915615869.
22. Krebs EE, Carey TS, Weinberger M. Accuracy of the pain numeric rating scale as a screening test in primary care. J Gen Intern Med. 2007;22(10):1453–8. https://doi.org/10.1007/s11606-007-0321-2.

23. Louw A, Diener I, Butler DS, Puentedura EJ. The effect of neuroscience education on pain, disability, anxiety, and stress in chronic musculoskeletal pain. Arch Phys Med Rehabil. 2011;92(12):2041–56. https://doi.org/10.1016/j.apmr.2011.07.198.
24. McGill University. The pain catastrophizing scale (PCS). Centre for Research on Pain, Disability and Social Integration. n.d. Retrieved May 5, 2025, from https://sullivan--painresearch.mcgill.ca/pcs.php
25. MD Anderson Cancer Center. Brief Pain Inventory (BPI). n.d. Retrieved May 5, 2025, from https://www.mdanderson.org/research/departments-labs-institutes/departments-divisions/symptom-research/symptom-assessment-tools/brief-pain-inventory.html
26. Mendell LM. Constructing and deconstructing the gate theory of pain. Pain. 2014;155(2):210–6. https://doi.org/10.1016/j.pain.2013.12.010.
27. Mendoza TR, Chen C, Brugger A, Hubbard R, Snabes M, Palmer SN, Zhang Q, Cleeland CS. The utility and validity of the modified brief pain inventory in a multiple-dose postoperative analgesic trial. Clin J Pain. 2004;20(5):357–62. https://doi.org/10.1097/00002508-200409000-00011.
28. Mills SEE, Nicolson KP, Smith BH. Chronic pain: a review of its epidemiology and associated factors in population-based studies. Br J Anaesth. 2019;123(2):e273–83. https://doi.org/10.1016/j.bja.2019.03.023.
29. Mills S, Torrance N, Smith BH. Identification and management of chronic pain in primary care: a review. Curr Psychiatry Rep. 2016;18(2):22. https://doi.org/10.1007/s11920-015-0659-9.
30. Monticone M, Baiardi P, Ferrari S, Foti C, Mugnai R, Pillastrini P, Rocca B, Vanti C. Development of the Italian version of the Pain Catastrophising Scale (PCS-I): cross-cultural adaptation, factor analysis, reliability, validity and sensitivity to change. Qual Life Res. 2012;21(6):1045–50. https://doi.org/10.1007/s11136-011-0007-4.
31. Morales ME, Yong RJ. Racial and ethnic disparities in the treatment of chronic pain. Pain Med. 2021;22(1):75–90. https://doi.org/10.1093/pm/pnaa427.
32. Moseley GL, Butler DS. Fifteen years of explaining pain: the past, present, and future. J Pain. 2015;16(9):807–13. https://doi.org/10.1016/j.jpain.2015.05.005.
33. Niknejad B, Bolier R, Henderson CR Jr, Delgado D, Kozlov E, Löckenhoff CE, Reid MC. Association between psychological interventions and chronic pain outcomes in older adults: a systematic review and meta-analysis. JAMA Intern Med. 2018;178(6):830–9. https://doi.org/10.1001/jamainternmed.2018.0756.
34. Osman A, Barrios FX, Gutierrez PM, Kopper BA, Merrifield T, Grittmann L. The pain catastrophizing scale: further psychometric evaluation with adult samples. J Behav Med. 2000;23(4):351–65. https://doi.org/10.1023/A:1005548801037.
35. Overstreet DS, Pester BD, Wilson JM, Flowers KM, Kline NK, Meints SM. The experience of BIPOC living with chronic pain in the USA: biopsychosocial factors that underlie racial disparities in pain outcomes, comorbidities, inequities, and barriers to treatment. Curr Pain Headache Rep. 2023;27(1):1–10. https://doi.org/10.1007/s11916-022-01098-8.
36. Padua L, Briani C, Truini A, Aprile I, Bouhassirà D, Cruccu G, Jann S, Nobile-Orazio E, Pazzaglia C, Morini A, Mondelli M, Ciaramitaro P, Cavaletti G, Cocito D, Fazio R, Santoro L, Galeotti F, Carpo M, Plasmati R, et al. Consistence and discrepancy of neuropathic pain screening tools DN4 and ID-pain. Neurol Sci. 2013;34(3):373–7. https://doi.org/10.1007/s10072-012-1011-3.
37. Paultre K, Cade W, Hernandez D, Reynolds J, Greif D, Best TM. Therapeutic effects of turmeric or curcumin extract on pain and function for individuals with knee osteoarthritis: a systematic review. BMJ Open Sport Exerc Med. 2021;7(1):e000935. https://doi.org/10.1136/bmjsem-2020-000935.
38. Portenoy R. Development and testing of a neuropathic pain screening questionnaire: ID pain. Curr Med Res Opin. 2006;22(8):1555–65. https://doi.org/10.1185/030079906X115702.
39. Quartana PJ, Campbell CM, Edwards RR. Pain catastrophizing: a critical review. Expert Rev Neurother. 2009;9(5):745–58. https://doi.org/10.1586/ERN.09.34.

40. Reyes-Gibby C, Morrow PK, Bennett MI, Jensen MP, Shete S. Neuropathic pain in breast cancer survivors: using the ID Pain as a screening tool. J Pain Symptom Manag. 2010;39(5):882–9. https://doi.org/10.1016/j.jpainsymman.2009.09.020.
41. Rowbotham MC. What is a 'clinically meaningful' reduction in pain? Pain. 2001;94(2):131–2. https://doi.org/10.1016/S0304-3959(01)00371-2.
42. Scott EL, Kroenke K, Wu J, Yu Z. Beneficial effects of improvement in depression, pain catastrophizing, and anxiety on pain outcomes: a 12-month longitudinal analysis. J Pain. 2016;17(2):215–22. https://doi.org/10.1016/j.jpain.2015.10.011.
43. Seal K, Becker W, Tighe J, Li Y, Rife T. Managing chronic pain in primary care: it really does take a village. J Gen Intern Med. 2017;32(8):931–4. https://doi.org/10.1007/s11606-017-4047-5.
44. Shavers VL, Bakos A, Sheppard VB. Race, ethnicity, and pain among the U.S. adult population. J Health Care Poor Underserved. 2010;21(1):177–220. https://doi.org/10.1353/hpu.0.0255.
45. Sielski R, Rief W, Glombiewski JA. Efficacy of biofeedback in chronic back pain: a meta-analysis. Int J Behav Med. 2017;24(1):25–41. https://doi.org/10.1007/s12529-016-9572-9.
46. Song C-Y, Lin S-F, Huang C-Y, Wu H-C, Chen C-H, Hsieh C-L. Validation of the brief pain inventory in patients with low back pain. Spine. 2016;41(15):E937. https://doi.org/10.1097/BRS.0000000000001478.
47. Sönmez DZ, Taşcı S. The effect of St. John's Wort oil (Hypericum Perforatum L.) in knee osteoarthritis: a randomized controlled and qualitative study. Pain Manag Nurs. 2024;25(2):e115–25. https://doi.org/10.1016/j.pmn.2023.12.002.
48. Stanos S, Brodsky M, Argoff C, Clauw DJ, D'Arcy Y, Donevan S, Gebke KB, Jensen MP, Lewis & Clark E, McCarberg B, Park PW, Turk DC, Watt S. Rethinking chronic pain in a primary care setting. Postgrad Med. 2016;128(5):502–15. https://doi.org/10.1080/00325481.2016.1188319.
49. Stephens K, Raue P (Directors). Brief behavioral skills: behavioral activation [Video]. Youtube. 2019. https://youtu.be/fqk41YZ81uM?si=aOc4VpBqqTDVjM11.
50. Sullivan MJL, Bishop SR, Pivik J. The pain catastrophizing scale: development and validation. Psychol Assess. 1995;7(4):524–32. https://doi.org/10.1037/1040-3590.7.4.524.
51. Sullivan MJL, Tripp DA. Pain catastrophizing: controversies, misconceptions and future directions. J Pain. 2024;25(3):575–87. https://doi.org/10.1016/j.jpain.2023.07.004.
52. Tan G, Jensen MP, Thornby JI, Shanti BF. Validation of the brief pain inventory for chronic nonmalignant pain. J Pain. 2004;5(2):133–7. https://doi.org/10.1016/j.jpain.2003.12.005.
53. Therapeutic Research Center. Natural medicines comprehensive database. 2024. https://naturalmedicines.therapeuticresearch.com.
54. Treede R-D, Rief W, Barke A, Aziz Q, Bennett MI, Benoliel R, Cohen M, Evers S, Finnerup NB, First MB, Giamberardino MA, Kaasa S, Korwisi B, Kosek E, Lavand'homme P, Nicholas M, Perrot S, Scholz J, Schug S, et al. Chronic pain as a symptom or a disease: the IASP classification of chronic pain for the International Classification of Diseases (ICD-11). Pain. 2019;160(1):19. https://doi.org/10.1097/j.pain.0000000000001384.
55. Vargas AJ, Tobey-Moore L, Curran GM, Elkhateb R, Sexton KW, Bailey BJ, Nagel C, Goree JH. Exploring racial disparities in chronic pain management. J Pain Res. 2025;18:2901–8. https://doi.org/10.2147/JPR.S493664.
56. Yang C-C, Ro L-S, Tsai Y-C, Lin K-P, Sun W-Z, Fang W-T, Wang S-J. Development and validation of a Taiwan version of the ID Pain questionnaire (ID Pain-T). J Chin Med Assoc. 2018;81(1):12–7. https://doi.org/10.1016/j.jcma.2017.06.019.
57. Yap JC, Lau J, Chen PP, Gin T, Wong T, Chan I, Chu J, Wong E. Validation of the Chinese Pain Catastrophizing Scale (HK-PCS) in patients with chronic pain. Pain Med. 2008;9(2):186–95. https://doi.org/10.1111/j.1526-4637.2007.00307.x.

Chapter 7
Irritable Bowel Syndrome

Kimberly A. Muellers, Stella D. Nelms, and Molly A. Warren

Case Vignette

Mr. C is a 36-year-old male presenting to establish care. He has a history of anxiety, constipation, and diarrhea.

Mr. C*: I'm worried I have cancer or celiac disease. I get constipated every time I travel. Sometimes I cannot poop for days, I feel bloated, I have gas, and it hurts when I finally poop. I have abdominal pain and diarrhea, like before a big presentation at work.*

Dr. W: *You're worried about having something serious, like cancer. Have you ever brought this up with another doctor?*

Mr. C*: Last year I had a colonoscopy and endoscopy. I was told everything was "normal." But I don't feel normal. Do you think I have cancer?*

Dr. W: *If both colonoscopy and endoscopy were normal, it's unlikely that you have cancer. Have you noticed anything that helps or worsens your symptoms?*

Mr. C: *Eating vegetables and drinking water helps with constipation. Diarrhea happens when I'm nervous, like before work presentations or going to a party where I don't know many people. Then once I go to the bathroom, my stomach pain goes away.*

K. A. Muellers (✉)
Department of Psychology, The New School for Social Research, New York, NY, USA

Department of Psychology, Pace University, New York, NY, USA
e-mail: kmuellers@pace.edu

S. D. Nelms
Division of Neuropsychology and Behavioral Health, Department of Rehabilitation Medicine, Emory University School of Medicine, Atlanta, GA, USA

M. A. Warren
Direct Primary Care and Acupuncture, Bentleyville, OH, USA

N. Pilipenko, K. M. Desai (eds.), *8 Conditions Primary Care Clinicians Dread to Treat*, https://doi.org/10.1007/978-3-032-12819-5_7

Dr. W: *I see how distressing this is. Based on your symptoms—abdominal pain that gets better with bowel movement, as well as constipation, diarrhea—your symptoms meet criteria for* ***irritable bowel syndrome (IBS)****.*

Mr. C: *I've heard of* ***IBS****. Is it dangerous? Can it be cured?*

Dr. W: ***IBS*** *is not dangerous. It is a chronic condition, so it cannot be "cured" but you can learn to manage it over time. Good news is that with the right tools, you can definitely feel better. To pick the best approach, we need to understand your triggers. I want you to keep a daily log of your food intake, symptoms, timing and frequency of bowel movement for two weeks. We will review it together at our next visit.*

Mr. C: *I have to track everything I eat? That sounds annoying. How will this help me?*

Dr. W: *I get it—tracking can feel like a hassle at first. Some people find that using an app can help. It will allow us to better understand your symptoms since* ***IBS*** *affects everybody differently. It will help us tailor your treatment. This is a temporary strategy, but it's important that you track daily to make sure that we have a full picture.*

Mr. C: *Ok, I'll try.*

Mr. C was scheduled for one-month follow-up. The following laboratory tests were ordered to rule out inflammatory bowel disease and celiac disease: full blood count, erythrocyte sedimentation rate, C-reactive protein, endomysial antibodies, and tissue transglutaminase. Dr. W also asks Mr. C to watch an educational video about **IBS** prior to the next visit (Resources: HealthSketch).

Diagnosis: Brief Description

The autonomic nervous system plays a major role in **IBS**, thus it is known as a disorder of **gut-brain interaction** (DGBI; [17]). **IBS** is characterized by abdominal pain and abnormal stool frequency and/or consistency [6]. The Rome IV criteria classify **IBS** sub-types and provide the gold standard for **IBS** diagnosis [43]. While the optimal path from identifying to treating **IBS** is subject to an ongoing debate, current guidelines suggest that **IBS** can be diagnosed based on patient-reported symptoms [6]. However, additional testing is recommended when "alarm" symptoms indicating inflammatory bowel disease (IBD) or cancer are present (See [35] for details). Furthermore, celiac disease and bacterial overgrowth should be ruled out or managed before diagnosing **IBS** [6].

Diagnosis of this multifaceted condition should involve a physical exam, collection of medical history, examination of a stool sample and/or description using the Bristol Stool Form Scale [10], and patient-reported symptom assessment.

Prevalence, Risk Factors, and Disparities

IBS affects 11% of the global population and 7–16% of the U.S. population [11], however precise prevalence is unknown [12]. In primary care (PC), **IBS** is likely underdetected, as only 10–50% of patients with **IBS** seek medical care [12].

IBS is more commonly diagnosed in females than males (14% vs. 8.9%), though this discrepancy may reflect sociocultural differences in care-seeking [11]. Furthermore, half of **IBS** cases begin before age 35, and symptoms typically decrease in older age [12].

In the U.S., **IBS** is more frequently diagnosed among White and Asian individuals compared with Black and Hispanic/Latino populations [13]. This is attributed to a combination of cultural factors and underdiagnosis due to disparities in healthcare access and utilization [13]. Racial/ethnic minority patients with **IBS** receive fewer GI consults, undergo more GI procedures, and pay higher emergency care costs [48, 49]. Unfortunately, mechanisms underlying these discrepancies are not well understood. It is unknown if these differences represent provider bias, miscommunication, or patient preferences, highlighting the need for further research [44].

IBS is multifactorial in origin [17]. Contributors include genetic factors, diet, gut microbiome composition, low-grade inflammation, neuroendocrine disturbances, heightened **visceral sensitivity (VS)**, abnormal gut motility, childhood abuse, and parental reinforcement [30]. Approximately 35–45% of **IBS** cases are post-infectious, developing following acute gastroenteritis [30]. Moreover, chemical irritants can trigger **IBS** through bacterial overgrowth/imbalance [11]. **IBS** is highly comorbid with other GI conditions, non-GI conditions of unclear organic origin (e.g. fibromyalgia, chronic fatigue), anxiety, and depression [13].

Symptom Assessment Tools

Table 7.1 presents three validated **IBS** tools. The **IBS** Severity Scoring System uses five visual analog items to estimate current **IBS** symptom severity [21]. The Gastrointestinal Symptom Rating Scale for IBS provides an open-access option for measuring discomfort due to **IBS** symptoms [54]. The IBS Quality of Life scale can aid in assessment of key psychosocial aspects of **IBS** [39].

In addition to these **IBS**-specific measures, the literature supports the utility of general pain assessment tools to measure **IBS**-related pain. Specifically, the Short-form McGill Pain Questionnaire [19] can assess pain-related beliefs and distress via the Pain Catastrophizing Scale [51]. Findings should be interpreted in the context of other, **IBS**-specific data [36]. Furthermore, the Digestive Symptoms and Impact Questionnaire and the Gastrointestinal Symptoms Severity Index may be useful if a patient presents with symptoms fitting criteria for more than one GI condition [16, 53].

Table 7.1 IBS screening tools

Screener Name	Items #	Rating scale scoring	Cut offs	Assessment timeline	Availability	Psychometric properties	Non-English versions available?
Irritable Bowel Severity Scoring System (IBSSS)	5 [21]	Visual scale [21] 0–100 [21]	≥75—concern for IBS 75–175—mild 175–300—moderate >300—severe [21]	10 days [21]	Copyrighted [55]	Good discriminant validity from controls and IBS in remission Good test-retest reliability within 24 h Good sensitivity to change [21]	Arabic [1], Spanish [2]
Gastrointestinal Symptom Rating Scale for IBS (GSRS-IBS)	13 [54]	7-point Likert [54] 1 = No discomfort at all to 7 = Very severe discomfort [54]	No established cutoffs	1 week [54]	Open access [3]	Good internal consistency and construct validity [54] High convergent and divergent validity [33]	None
IBS Quality of Life (IBS-QOL)	34 [56]	5-point Likert [56] 1 = Not at all to 5 = Extremely/a great deal [56]	No established cutoffs	1 month [56]	Copyrighted [46]	High internal consistency (Cronbach's $\alpha = 0.95$) and reproducibility (ICC = 0.86) [56] Significant convergent validity [18] Effective discriminant validity [18]	Chinese [27], Spanish [45]

Non-pharmacological Conceptualization: What to Say to the Patient?

Discussing **IBS** using a **biopsychosocial (BPS)** approach is an important albeit challenging task. The following section presents key messages to relay to patients about **IBS**.

Message #1: Understanding and Managing IBS Requires a BPS Perspective

The human gut functions in coordination with the brain. What this means is that thoughts and feelings affect the gut. **IBS** symptoms can be worse during times of stress, while having worse GI symptoms can also cause stress and anxiety. Unfortunately, sometimes the brain and gut become overly sensitive to each other's signals. This leads to problems with gut functioning and produces **IBS** symptoms. While **IBS** symptoms are distressing and get in the way of functioning, they do not cause damage and are not dangerous. However, it is very common that specific situations, times, or places trigger **IBS** symptoms. Once **IBS** pain and discomfort emerge, these can affect wellbeing. Thus the brain and gut become more interconnected.

In order to manage **IBS**, different strategies and tools can be used to target the gut, brain and their communication. These tools include medication, diet, stress management, and trigger identification and modification.

Why? Physicians describe **IBS** as "moderately to extremely difficult to treat effectively" [24]. This might be due to misalignment between physicians' goals (excluding organic disease) and patients' goals (symptom relief) as well as physicians' focus on the biomedical model. Ignoring psychosocial aspects of **IBS** can lead to higher healthcare use, more severe symptoms, and poorer treatment response [38]. Moreover, misconceptions about **IBS**' causes and consequences are common. Research indicates that 30% of patients with **IBS** reported belief that **IBS** increased IBD risk, and 14% believed **IBS** could lead to GI cancer [7]. Such concerns may increase distress leading to ongoing requests for diagnostic and exploratory procedures.

To address these issues, effective **IBS** management requires BPS conceptualization [31] which should be explained clearly to the patient. Eliciting patient concerns and providing information early in the relationship builds trust and mutual understanding (see Vignette for demonstration).

Message #2: Setting Realistic Goals Is Key to IBS Treatment Success

Unfortunately, at this point no cure for **IBS** is available. However it is possible to decrease interference of **IBS** symptoms with goals and activities. Such goals can include: decreased symptom frequency, less pain, less distress, and/or ongoing participation in activities (see Vignette for example). Improved symptoms control requires a period of symptom tracking as well as trying various interventions. Over time, improved understanding of both triggers and management strategies will lead to better symptom control and less suffering.

Why? Setting realistic expectations and goals is crucial to **IBS** treatment. Patients with **IBS** report high levels of frustration and dissatisfaction with care [7]. Being transparent with patients about treatment expectations and eliciting their questions and concerns can alleviate frustration. Targeting the patient's most upsetting symptoms can provide earlier relief, reducing distress and increasing satisfaction with care [7].

Case Vignette, Continued

Mr. C returns for follow-up to discuss his diagnosis and treatment options after four weeks.

Dr. W*: Today I would like to go over the results of your bloodwork, review the information I sent you about* ***IBS****, and your symptom diary, and set some goals for treatment together. First, your blood work showed that you do not have IBD or celiac disease. Do you have any questions about this?*

Mr. C: *No, that's good to hear.*

Dr. W: *Great. Next, I want to make sure the materials I sent you were clear about what* ***IBS*** *is. What was your understanding of* ***IBS****?*

Mr. C: *The video said our brain and our gut communicate, but sometimes, these signals can get all confused and overly sensitive.*

Dr. W: *I think you are bringing up the key mechanism of* ***IBS*** *which unfortunately makes it so hard to manage it. Also* ***IBS*** *is a chronic condition which can take time to manage. Now let's review your two-week symptom diary. How did that go for you?*

Mr. C*: I liked the app. It was informational and easy to use. There were foods that triggered gas, bloating, and diarrhea. Steak and onions made it worse one night and then chili did a few days later.*

Dr. W: *The tracking is clearly showing that those are triggers for you. Is there anything you think these foods have in common?*

Mr. C: Yes, the app also discussed that foods high in certain sugars can trigger ***IBS*** *symptoms, and I saw that onions and beans have high sugars.*

Dr. W: That's right: foods high in some types of sugar, called ***FODMAP****s, are harder to digest. These can trigger* ***IBS*** *symptoms—onions, garlic, and beans are common culprits, which you noticed.* [See IM section for further details on **FODMAPS**s]. *What are some short-term goals you would like to set for your* ***IBS****?*

Mr. C: I have a presentation for work at the end of next week. I don't want to have diarrhea around the time of the presentation.

Dr. W: Let's see what can be possible. Can we look at your symptom diary again? How did stress impact your bowel movements?

*Mr. C: While I was tracking my symptoms, I had a performance review at work. I had diarrhea immediately before. I get it now, that's probably stress triggering my **IBS** symptoms. I just don't know how to stop feeling stressed.*

Dr. W: We may not be able to stop the causes of stress, but there are definitely ways to better manage your body's stress. Can we review a relaxation technique together?

Mr. C: *Sure.*

Dr. W proceeded to lead Mr. C through a progressive muscle relaxation [See Resources: Norelli 2025].

Non-pharmacological Treatment Options: What Can Be Done?

1. **Monitoring Triggers Is Essential for Improved Symptom Control**

What is it? Diet and physical activity changes are important initial techniques to promote **IBS** symptom control [32]. Most patients associate their **IBS** symptoms with eating meals and/or with intake of specific foods, typically carbohydrates [14]. However, **IBS** symptoms can change over time and patients often struggle to identify triggers that could be the target of lifestyle interventions. Thus, tracking of **IBS** symptoms along with possible triggers (e.g. foods, medications, stress) is essential to effective treatment.

How to address? First, clear communication about the role of lifestyle changes in **IBS** treatment can increase patient buy-in, improving adherence, autonomy, and self-efficacy [28]. Patients diagnosed with **IBS** should be instructed to keep a diary of all food eaten and IBS symptoms for a minimum of 3 days to identify diet-related triggers [14]. Physicians should provide patients with electronic or pen-and-paper tracking tools depending on individual preference and technological literacy (see Resources). Tracking data should be collaboratively reviewed together to identify triggers and management strategies. If the patient does not complete tracking, review the purpose of tracking and its importance for treatment planning. Engage patients in problem-solving around any barriers.

2. **Educate About Connections Between IBS- Related Thoughts, Feeling and Behaviors and Teach Relevant Techniques**

What is it? Patients' perceptions of symptoms (especially catastrophic beliefs about risks and lack of control) play a significant role in **IBS** outcomes [47]. Figure 7.1 presents cognitive-behavioral conceptualization illustrating links between symptoms. Repetition of these thoughts, emotions, and behaviors can increase autonomic nervous system arousal, in turn worsening **IBS** symptoms.

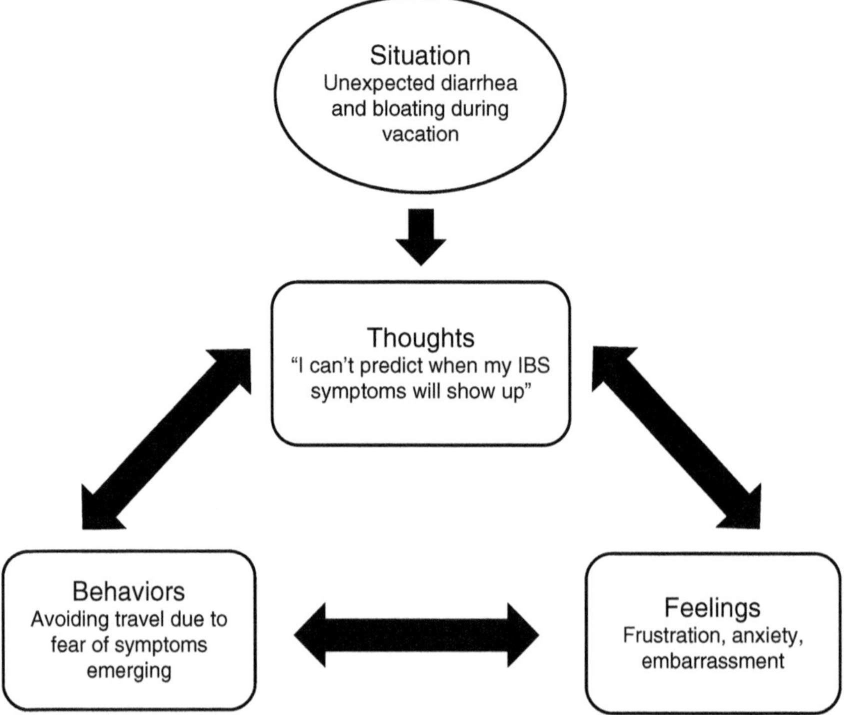

Fig. 7.1 Cognitive-behavioral triangle example

How to address? *Cognitive disputation* can help patients recognize unhelpful thoughts and replace them with more balanced, helpful thinking. For detailed discussion, see Chap. 2.

Another strategy is to teach patients *worry management* using Stimulus Control Training (SCT). Engaging in this process daily leads the designated worry time/place to become a cue for worry, while other cues weaken [28], allowing the patient increased control over catastrophic thinking and **IBS** symptoms. For detailed instructions on SCT, please see Chap. 2.

3. **Teach Techniques to Improve VS**

What is it? VS is a key mechanism of **IBS** in which normal gut activity becomes interpreted as dangerous and/or the gut reacts abnormally to brain signals [25]. Changes in **VS** may maintain the relationship between triggers and symptoms in **IBS** while interventions targeting this mechanism can lead to symptom relief [6].

How to address?

VS can be altered through interventions which promote relaxation, including: diaphragmatic breathing, progressive muscle relaxation, and mindfulness practice [50], relieving symptoms and improving quality of life [26].

Following are instructions for a relaxing breathing exercise:

- Take a normal breath in through your nose with your mouth closed. Pause for a moment.
- As you exhale, make an "O" with your mouth and slowly let all the air out of your lungs. Silently say to yourself a word like "calm" or "relax".
- Pause again, then take the next breath in.
- Focus on slow breaths rather than deep breaths. Use your belly to breathe, rather than your chest.
- Continue breathing in this manner and count your inhales and exhales up to 10. If you get distracted, gently bring yourself back to the exercise and restart at 1. The goal is not to reach 10, but to keep returning your thoughts to your breath.

Additional options for targeting **VS** are included under Resources.

Psychotherapy Effectiveness

Physicians may consider referral to psychotherapy if a patient's **IBS** symptoms are refractory, defined in **IBS** as failure of symptom resolution via medication and lifestyle modifications after 12 months of treatment [30].

A meta-analysis of randomized controlled trials (RCTs) testing psychotherapy for **IBS** found that cognitive behavioral therapy (CBT; self-administered: risk ratio [RR] = .61, 95% CI = .45–.83; face-to-face: RR = .62, 95% CI = .48–.80) and gut-directed hypnotherapy (RR = 0.67, 95% CI = .49–.91) effectively reduce patient-reported **IBS** symptoms [9]. A network meta-analysis similarly found reduced or resolved abdominal symptoms (self-administered CBT: RR = .71, 95% CI = .54–.95; face-to-face CBT: RR = .72, 95% CI = .54–.97; gut-directed hypnotherapy : RR = .77, 95% CI = .61–.96; [23]). Group-based CBT was also more effective than routine care [23].

CBT can reduce **IBS** symptoms, improve quality of life, and lessen psychological distress by changing illness-specific cognitions, anxiety, and behaviors [41], with evidence for both short-term [52] and long-term effectiveness, particularly among patients with refractory symptoms [20]. "Minimal contact" (≤4 sessions) and self-directed CBT show large effects in reducing **IBS** symptoms [9]. One study demonstrated clinically meaningful **IBS** symptom reductions (IBS-SSS score change ≥50) in 71% of patients receiving telephone-based CBT and 63% receiving web-based CBT, compared to 46% receiving treatment-as-usual [20].

Mindfulness-focused interventions show promise for **IBS** treatment, with one RCT reporting a 38.2% reduction in **IBS** symptom severity, reduced psychological distress, and improved quality of life following an 8-week intervention [4].

Gut-directed hypnotherapy combines physical relaxation, GI-focused relaxation, metaphors, and suggestion [37] and can reduce pain, bloating, and bowel dysfunction and improve quality of life in 7–10 sessions [4]. While the mechanisms of gut-directed hypnotherapy are not fully understood, it may alter **visceral sensitivity** by training patients to attend to and modify **gut-brain interactions** [4]. There is evidence that hypnotherapy improves **IBS** symptoms in the short- and long-term [52], with 83% of responders in one study maintaining improvements 1–5 years post-treatment [22]. Gut-directed hypnotherapy can be delivered individually or in groups [9].

Brief psychodynamic psychotherapy may also be effective for **IBS** management [4]. In one study, health-related quality-of-life improved by 5.2 points among **IBS** patients receiving therapy compared to 5.8 points for paroxetine and −.3 points for treatment-as-usual [15]. However, studies of psychodynamic therapy for **IBS** remain limited.

Despite this evidence, current American College of Gastroenterology guidelines only conditionally support CBT and gut-directed hypnotherapy in **IBS** due to limitations of the existing literature [32]. Many RCTs to date have tested psychotherapy only as an adjunctive treatment for **IBS**, and trials often do not restrict pharmacotherapy use; therefore, the effectiveness of psychotherapy alone is not well understood [32]. Thus, while CBT and hypnotherapy for **IBS** are considered low-risk and potentially beneficial, referrals should be given with the limitations of the research in mind.

Integrative Medicine Interventions and Techniques

Dietary Modifications: FODMAP

FODMAPs (Fermentable Oligo-, Di-, Mono-saccharides, And Polyols) are poorly absorbed carbohydrates, which increase gastrointestinal water secretion and fermentation. Common, high-**FODMAP** foods include cruciferous vegetables, wheat, dairy, beans, lentils, and fruits such as apples and pears. The American Gastroenterology Association (AGA) recommends a low-**FODMAP** diet for **IBS** as a first-line approach [14]. A meta-analysis findings report 33% symptom reduction associated with low-**FODMAP** diet [8]. Under the guidance of a dietician or nutritionist, a low-**FODMAP** diet can be personalized to each patient, promoting an individualized approach to symptom management.

Physical Activity

The AGA recommends exercise for improvement in **IBS** symptoms [6]. Specifically, walking 60 min per day, three days per week was found to reduce severity of abdominal pain by 48.6%, frequency of abdominal pain by 60.4%, and severity of bloating by 39.2% [42]. Walking is a safe and accessible exercise that physicians can recommend for many patients with **IBS**.

Herbs/Botanicals/Supplements

Overall, the current evidence for supplements in **IBS** is of low quality.

Psyllium

Psyllium is a soluble fiber that can be especially helpful for patients with constipation-predominant **IBS**. By absorbing water, **psyllium** adds bulk to the stool, which firms stool in diarrhea-predominant and softens stool in constipation-predominant **IBS**. Daily addition of 10g of **psyllium** powder (in two doses) for 12 weeks resulted in adequate relief of abdominal pain for 57% patients receiving **psyllium** (RR = 1.60, 95% CI = 1.13–2.26), and a number needed to treat (NNT) of 4 [5]. **Psyllium** powder can be recommended to patients and can be mixed into water or foods such as yogurt.

Peppermint Oil

Using **peppermint oil** delivered in enteric coated capsules of 180-225 mg, 2–3 times per day over 4–8 weeks significantly improved abdominal pain in **IBS** compared with placebo. Patients taking **peppermint oil** were 24% less likely to have no improvement in abdominal pain (RR = .76; 95% CI = .62–.93), corresponding to a NNT of 7. Side effects, including heartburn and flatulence, were reported with **peppermint oil** [29].

Acupuncture

A 2012 Cochrane Review found that **acupuncture** produced greater improvement in IBS symptoms than two antispasmodic medications [34]. In an RCT of 531 patients, **acupuncture** (three sessions per week for 6 weeks) was compared with daily polyethylene glycol and pinaverium bromide. At 6 weeks, the **acupuncture** group showed greater IBS-SSS score reductions (−123.5 vs. −94.7). At 12-week follow-up, improvements in IBS-SSS (−127.2) and IBS-related quality of life (+16.2) remained significant compared to baseline and pharmacotherapy [40]. Physicians may refer patients to licensed **acupuncture** providers, and patients should verify insurance coverage.

Clinical Pearls

- Discuss **IBS** diagnosis from a BPS perspective and limit additional testing unless warranted by "alarm" symptoms.
- Discuss IBS as the consequence of disordered **gut-brain interaction**.
- Engage patients in symptoms and **trigger monitoring** to guide personalized **IBS** management.
- Assist patients in setting realistic expectations and goals for **IBS** management.
- Discuss the importance of lifestyle modifications including a low-**FODMAP** diet, moderate-intensity aerobic exercise, and stress management.
- Teach cognitive and/or relaxation skills to patients to address **VS**.
- Consider referring patients with severe or refractory **IBS** symptoms for gut-focused CBT or hypnotherapy.

Frequently Asked Questions

Question 1: *How can you be sure this is* ***IBS*** *and not something more serious? I feel like I should get a colonoscopy.*

Answer: Based on your symptoms, we can actually diagnose **IBS** without doing invasive testing, which will save us time and get you feeling better sooner. I will keep monitoring your lab values and symptoms, and if anything changes unexpectedly I can refer you to a gastroenterologist to make sure everything is okay.

Question 2: *I'm not sure about all these diet changes: it seems like a lot of work, and when I tried eating healthy in the past I still had issues. Can't I just take a pill?*

Answer: I understand lifestyle changes can be difficult, and it can be frustrating to hear that I want you to try these changes when you were hoping there would be a quicker solution. I am happy to discuss medications that could help relieve your symptoms when they happen, but making changes to your diet might mean that you need these medications less often. Maybe you can start by telling me a bit more about what your diet looked like when you were 'eating healthy,' and we can choose some small changes to make for now?

Question 3: *I'm just worried that I'll have symptoms at a really inconvenient time, like while I'm stuck in traffic or in a meeting. It feels like I'm always waiting for the worst to happen!*

Answer: **IBS** symptoms can be hard to predict or control. Identifying your triggers and making changes to your daily life should help make your symptoms more predictable over time.

Case Vignette: Conclusion

Mr. C returns in eight weeks for a follow-up.

Mr. C: *I am feeling a bit better. I started practicing progressive muscle relaxation at work, and it has helped with my anxiety. I gave a presentation without having diarrhea.*

Dr. W: *I'm happy to hear that. How has food been affecting your symptoms?*

Mr. C: *I still like to eat garlic and onions, but I notice if I eat less dairy and fewer beans my symptoms are better. I still get abdominal pain throughout the day. Is there something else I can take for this?*

Dr. W proceeds to discuss evidence for **psyllium** husk [see IM section]. They agree to follow-up in three months.

Resources

Source	Description	Link
Patient Education		
Irritable Bowel Syndrome.net	Website with psychoeducation, self-management resources, and moderated community forum	https://irritablebowelsyndrome.net/
HealthSketch	"What is IBS? (Irritable Bowel Syndrome)" Duration: 4:07	https://www.youtube.com/watch?v=Lk1wn0jjZR0
Osmosis by Elsevier	"Irritable bowel syndrome (IBS)—causes, symptoms, risk factors, treatment, pathology" Duration: 4:06	https://www.youtube.com/watch?v=E86eXpVBTcI
Cleveland Clinic	"What Is IBS? I Ask Cleveland Clinic's Expert" Duration: 3:38	https://www.youtube.com/watch?v=Qmze4Cb9N20
Self-guided tools and apps		
The Calm & Happy Gut	Gut-directed hypnosis and meditation	https://www.youtube.com/watch?v=Ru_0ACtDSCw
Bowelle	Mobile IBS symptom tracking app, available for iPhone, free with in-app purchases	https://bowelle.com/
MyIBS	Free mobile IBS symptom tracking app by the Canadian Digestive Health Foundation	https://apps.apple.com/us/app/myibs-symptom-health-diary/id1592757407

(continued)

Source	Description	Link
Resources for providers		
The Rome Foundation	Rome IV criteria for diagnosis of IBS and sub-types	https://theromefoundation.org/rome-iv/rome-iv-criteria/
Irritable Bowel Syndrome.net	Printable IBS food diary	https://irritablebowelsyndrome.net/living/food-journal-download
Chey, W. D., Eswaran, S., & Kurlander, J. (2015)	Patient-friendly summary of IBS diagnosis, symptoms, and treatment	https://jamanetwork.com/journals/jama/fullarticle/2174031
Norelli, S. K., Long, A., & Krepps, J. M. (2025)	Easy, evidence-based relaxation techniques & scripts	https://www.ncbi.nlm.nih.gov/books/NBK513238/
U.S. Veteran's Association	Provider guide to autogenic training	https://www.myhealth.va.gov/mhv-portal-web/ss20240708-manage-stress-self-guided-relaxation
Brown University	Relaxation resources	https://www.brownhealth.org/centers-services/behavioral-medicine-clinical-services/relaxation-training
Digital Therapeutics		
Mahana IBS	FDA-cleared tool delivering 3-month psychoeducation and gut-directed CBT program	https://www.mahanatx.com/
Regulora by metaMe Health	FDA-cleared device intended for 3-month treatment of IBS-related abdominal pain	https://www.regulora.ca/

References

1. AbdAllah AM, Sharafeddin MA. Subjective sleep quality among patients with irritable bowel syndrome attending outpatient clinic in Zagazig University Hospital. Egypt J Community Med. 2021;39(1):23–31.
2. Almansa C, García-Sanchez R, Barceló M, Díaz-Rubio M, Rey E. Translation, cultural adaptation and validation of a Spanish version of the Irritable Bowel Syndrome Severity Score. Rev Esp Enferm Dig. 2011;103:612–8.
3. AstraZeneca. Gastrointestinal patient reported outcomes. 2025. https://www.astrazeneca.com/patient-reported-outcomes/gastrointestinal.html.
4. Ballou S, Keefer L. Psychological interventions for irritable bowel syndrome and inflammatory bowel diseases. Clin Transl Gastroenterol. 2017;8(1):e214. https://doi.org/10.1038/ctg.2016.69.
5. Bijkerk CJ, de Wit NJ, Muris JW, Whorwell PJ, Knottnerus JA, Hoes AW. Soluble or insoluble fibre in irritable bowel syndrome in primary care? Randomised placebo controlled trial. BMJ. 2009;339:b3154. https://doi.org/10.1136/bmj.b3154.

6. Black CJ, Ford AC. An evidence-based update on the diagnosis and management of irritable bowel syndrome. Expert Rev Gastroenterol Hepatol. 2025;19(3):227–42. https://doi.org/10.1080/17474124.2025.2455586.
7. Black CJ, Ford AC. Best management of irritable bowel syndrome. Frontline Gastroenterol. 2021;12(4):303–15. https://doi.org/10.1136/flgastro-2019-101298.
8. Black CJ, Staudacher HM, Ford AC. Efficacy of a low FODMAP diet in irritable bowel syndrome: systematic review and network meta-analysis. Gut. 2022;71(6):1117–26. https://doi.org/10.1136/gutjnl-2021-325214.
9. Black CJ, Thakur ER, Houghton LA, Quigley EMM, Moayyedi P, Ford AC. Efficacy of psychological therapies for irritable bowel syndrome: systematic review and network meta-analysis. Gut. 2020;69(8):1441–51. https://doi.org/10.1136/gutjnl-2020-321191.
10. Blake MR, Raker JM, Whelan K. Validity and reliability of the Bristol Stool Form Scale in healthy adults and patients with diarrhoea-predominant irritable bowel syndrome. Aliment Pharmacol Ther. 2016;44(7):693–703. https://doi.org/10.1111/apt.13746.
11. Camilleri M. Diagnosis and treatment of irritable bowel syndrome: a review. JAMA. 2021;325(9):865–77. https://doi.org/10.1001/jama.2020.22532.
12. Canavan C, West J, Card T. The epidemiology of irritable bowel syndrome. Clin Epidemiol. 2014;6:71–80. https://doi.org/10.2147/CLEP.S40245.
13. Cheng K, Lee C, Garniene R, Cabral H, Weber HC. Epidemiology of irritable bowel syndrome in a large academic safety-net hospital. J Clin Med. 2024;13(5):Article 5. https://doi.org/10.3390/jcm13051314.
14. Chey WD, Hashash JG, Manning L, Chang L. AGA clinical practice update on the role of diet in irritable bowel syndrome: expert review. Gastroenterology. 2022;162(6):1737–1745.e5. https://doi.org/10.1053/j.gastro.2021.12.248.
15. Creed F, Fernandes L, Guthrie E, Palmer S, Ratcliffe J, Read N, Rigby C, Thompson D, Tomenson B. The cost-effectiveness of psychotherapy and paroxetine for severe irritable bowel syndrome. Gastroenterology. 2003;124:303–17. https://doi.org/10.1053/gast.2003.50055.
16. Crowell MD, Umar SB, Lacy BE, Jones MP, DiBaise JK, Talley NJ. Multi-dimensional gastrointestinal symptom severity index: validation of a brief GI symptom assessment tool. Dig Dis Sci. 2015;60(8):2270–9. https://doi.org/10.1007/s10620-015-3647-3.
17. Drossman DA. Functional gastrointestinal disorders: history, pathophysiology, clinical features, and Rome IV. Gastroenterology. 2016;150(6):1262–1279.e2. https://doi.org/10.1053/j.gastro.2016.02.032.
18. Drossman DA, Patrick DL, Whitehead WE, Toner BB, Diamant NE, Hu Y, Jia H, Bangdiwala SI. Further validation of the IBS-QOL: a disease-specific quality-of-life questionnaire. Am J Gastroenterol. 2000;95(4):999. https://doi.org/10.1111/j.1572-0241.2000.01941.x.
19. Dworkin RH, Turk DC, Revicki DA, Harding G, Coyne KS, Peirce-Sandner S, Bhagwat D, Everton D, Burke LB, Cowan P, Farrar JT, Hertz S, Max MB, Rappaport BA, Melzack R. Development and initial validation of an expanded and revised version of the Short-form McGill Pain Questionnaire (SF-MPQ-2). Pain. 2009;144(1):35–42. https://doi.org/10.1016/j.pain.2009.02.007.
20. Everitt HA, Landau S, O'Reilly G, Sibelli A, Hughes S, Windgassen S, Holland R, Little P, McCrone P, Bishop FL, Goldsmith K, Coleman N, Logan R, Chalder T, Moss-Morris R. Cognitive behavioural therapy for irritable bowel syndrome: 24-month follow-up of participants in the ACTIB randomised trial. Lancet Gastroenterol Hepatol. 2019;4(11):863–72. https://doi.org/10.1016/S2468-1253(19)30243-2.
21. Francis CY, Morris J, Whorwell PJ. The irritable bowel severity scoring system: a simple method of monitoring irritable bowel syndrome and its progress. Aliment Pharmacol Ther. 1997;11(2):395–402. https://doi.org/10.1046/j.1365-2036.1997.142318000.x.
22. Gonsalkorale WM, Miller V, Afzal A, Whorwell PJ. Long term benefits of hypnotherapy for irritable bowel syndrome. Gut. 2003;52:1623–9. https://doi.org/10.1136/gut.52.11.1623.
23. Goodoory VC, Khasawneh M, Thakur ER, Everitt HA, Gudleski GD, Lackner JM, Moss-Morris R, Simren M, Vasant DH, Moayyedi P, Black CJ, Ford AC. Effect of brain-gut behav-

ioral treatments on abdominal pain in irritable bowel syndrome: systematic review and network meta-analysis. Gastroenterology. 2024;167(5):934–943.e5. https://doi.org/10.1053/j.gastro.2024.05.010.

24. Heidelbaugh JJ, Hungin AP, Palsson OS, Anastasiou F, Agreus L, Fracasso P, Maaroos H-I, Matic JR, Mendive JM, Seifert B, Drossman DA. Perceptions and practices of primary care providers in Europe and the US in the diagnosis and treatment of irritable bowel syndrome: a multinational survey. Neurogastroenterol Motil. 2025;37(2):e14967. https://doi.org/10.1111/nmo.14967.
25. Holtmann GJ, Ford AC, Talley NJ. Pathophysiology of irritable bowel syndrome. Lancet Gastroenterol Hepatol. 2016;1(2):133–46. https://doi.org/10.1016/S2468-1253(16)30023-1.
26. Horn A, Stangl S, Parisi S, Bauer N, Roll J, Löffler C, Gágyor I, Haas K, Heuschmann PU, Langhorst J, Keil T. Systematic review with meta-analysis: stress-management interventions for patients with irritable bowel syndrome. Stress Health. 2023;39(4):694–707. https://doi.org/10.1002/smi.3226.
27. Huang W, Zhou F, Bushnell DM, Diakite C, Yang X. Cultural adaptation and application of the IBS–QOL in China: a disease-specific quality-of-life questionnaire. Qual Life Res. 2007;16(6):991–6. https://doi.org/10.1007/s11136-006-9141-9.
28. Hunter CL, Goodie JL, Oordt MS, Dobmeyer AC. Chapter 8: Irritable bowel syndrome. In: Integrated behavioral health in primary care. American Psychological Association; 2022.
29. Ingrosso MR, Ianiro G, Nee J, Lembo AJ, Moayyedi P, Black CJ, Ford AC. Systematic review and meta-analysis: efficacy of peppermint oil in irritable bowel syndrome. Aliment Pharmacol Ther. 2022;56(6):932–41. https://doi.org/10.1111/apt.17179.
30. Khanbhai A, Singh Sura D. Irritable bowel syndrome for primary care physicians. Br J Med Pract. 2013;6(2):a608.
31. Lackner JM, Blanchard EB. Chapter 8: Cognitive therapy for irritable bowel syndrome: improving clinical decision making and treatment efficiency through behavioral case formulation. In: Formulation and treatment in clinical health psychology. Routledge/Taylor & Francis Group; 2006.
32. Lacy BE, Pimentel M, Brenner DM, Chey WD, Keefer LA, Long MD, Moshiree B. ACG clinical guideline: management of irritable bowel syndrome. Am J Gastroenterol. 2021;116(1):17–44. https://doi.org/10.14309/ajg.0000000000001036.
33. Ljótsson B, Jones M, Talley NJ, Kjellström L, Agréus L, Andreasson A. Discriminant and convergent validity of the GSRS-IBS symptom severity measure for irritable bowel syndrome: a population study. United European Gastroenterol J. 2020;8(3):284–92. https://doi.org/10.1177/2050640619900577.
34. Manheimer E, Cheng K, Wieland LS, Min LS, Shen X, Berman BM, Lao L. Acupuncture for treatment of irritable bowel syndrome. Cochrane Database Syst Rev. 2012;2012(5):CD005111. https://doi.org/10.1002/14651858.CD005111.pub3.
35. Moshiree B, Heidelbaugh JJ, Sayuk GS. A narrative review of irritable bowel syndrome with diarrhea: a primer for primary care providers. Adv Ther. 2022;39(9):4003–20. https://doi.org/10.1007/s12325-022-02224-z.
36. Mujagic Z, Keszthelyi D, Aziz Q, Reinisch W, Quetglas EG, De Leonardis F, Segerdahl M, Masclee AAM. Systematic review: instruments to assess abdominal pain in irritable bowel syndrome. Aliment Pharmacol Ther. 2015;42(9):1064–81. https://doi.org/10.1111/apt.13378.
37. Naliboff BD, Fresé MP, Rapgay L. Mind/body psychological treatments for irritable bowel syndrome. Evid Based Complement Alternat Med. 2008;5(1):919413. https://doi.org/10.1093/ecam/nem046.
38. Palsson OS, Drossman DA. Psychiatric and psychological dysfunction in irritable bowel syndrome and the role of psychological treatments. Gastroenterol Clin. 2005;34(2):281–303. https://doi.org/10.1016/j.gtc.2005.02.004.
39. Patrick DL, Drossman DA, Frederick IO, DiCesare J, Puder KL. Quality of life in persons with irritable bowel syndrome: development of a new measure. Dig Discovery Sci. 1998;43:400–11. https://doi.org/10.1023/A:1018831127942.

40. Pei L, Geng H, Guo J, Yang G, Wang L, Shen R, Xia S, Ding M, Feng H, Lu J, Li J, Liu L, Shu Y, Fang X, Wu X, Wang X, Weng S, Ju L, Chen X, Shen H, et al. Effect of acupuncture in patients with irritable bowel syndrome: a randomized controlled trial. Mayo Clin Proc. 2020;95(8):1671–83. https://doi.org/10.1016/j.mayocp.2020.01.042.
41. Radu M, Moldovan R, Pintea S, Băban A, Dumitraşcu D. Predictors of outcome in cognitive and behavioural interventions for irritable bowel syndrome. A meta-analysis. J Gastrointestin Liver Dis. 2018;27(3):Article 3. https://doi.org/10.15403/jgld.2014.1121.273.bab.
42. Riezzo G, Prospero L, D'Attoma B, Ignazzi A, Bianco A, Franco I, Curci R, Campanella A, Bonfiglio C, Osella AR, Russo F. The impact of a twelve-week moderate aerobic exercise program on gastrointestinal symptom profile and psychological well-being of irritable bowel syndrome patients: preliminary data from a southern Italy cohort. J Clin Med. 2023;12(16):5359. https://doi.org/10.3390/jcm12165359.
43. Rome Foundation. Rome IV Criteria. Rome Foundation; 2021. https://theromefoundation.org/rome-iv/rome-iv-criteria/.
44. Sasegbon A, Vasant DH. Understanding racial disparities in the care of patients with irritable bowel syndrome: the need for a unified approach. Neurogastroenterol Motil. 2021;33(5):e14152. https://doi.org/10.1111/nmo.14152.
45. Schmulson M, Ortiz O, Mejia-Arangure JM, Hu YB, Morris C, Arcila D, Gutierrez-Reyes G, Bangdiwala S, Drossman DA. Further validation of the IBS-QOL: female Mexican IBS patients have poorer quality of life than females from North Carolina. Dig Dis Sci. 2007;52(11):2950–5. https://doi.org/10.1007/s10620-006-9689-9.
46. Seattle Quality of Life Group. Irritable Bowel Syndrome Quality of Life Instrument (IBS-QOL). 2011. https://depts.washington.edu/seaqol/IBSQOL.
47. Sherwin LB, Leary E, Henderson WA. The association of catastrophizing with quality-of-life outcomes in patients with irritable bowel syndrome. Qual Life Res. 2017;26(8):2161–70. https://doi.org/10.1007/s11136-017-1554-0.
48. Shin A, Sarnoff R, Church A, Xu H, Chang L. The impact and interactions of race and gender on healthcare use and spending in irritable bowel syndrome. Clin Gastroenterol Hepatol. 2024; https://doi.org/10.1016/j.cgh.2024.11.005.
49. Silvernale C, Kuo B, Staller K. Racial disparity in healthcare utilization among patients with irritable bowel syndrome: results from a multicenter cohort. Neurogastroenterol Motil. 2021;33(5):e14039. https://doi.org/10.1111/nmo.14039.
50. Staudacher HM, Black CJ, Teasdale SB, Mikocka-Walus A, Keefer L. Irritable bowel syndrome and mental health comorbidity—approach to multidisciplinary management. Nat Rev Gastroenterol Hepatol. 2023;20(9):582–96. https://doi.org/10.1038/s41575-023-00794-z.
51. Sullivan MJL, Bishop SR, Pivik J. The pain catastrophizing scale: development and validation. Psychol Assess. 1995;7(4):524–32. https://doi.org/10.1037/1040-3590.7.4.524.
52. Surdea-Blaga T, Baban A, Nedelcu L, Dumitrascu DL. Psychological interventions for irritable bowel syndrome. J Gastrointestin Liver Dis. 2016;25(3):3. https://doi.org/10.15403/jgld.2014.1121.253.ibs.
53. Urnes J, Johannessen T, Farup PG, Stian L, Petersen H. Digestive symptoms and their psychosocial impact: validation of a questionnaire. Scand J Gastroenterol. 2006;41(9):1019–27. https://doi.org/10.1080/00365520600587402.
54. Wiklund IK, Fullerton S, Hawkey CJ, Jones RH, Longstreth GF, Mayer EA, Peacock RA, Wilson IK, Naesdal J. An irritable bowel syndrome-specific symptom questionnaire: development and validation. Scand J Gastroenterol. 2003;38(9):947–54. https://doi.org/10.1080/00365520310004209.
55. Rome Foundation. Copyright and licensing. 2021. https://theromefoundation.org/products/copyright-and-licensing/.
56. Patrick DL, Drossman DA, Frederick IO, DiCesare J, Puder KL. Quality of life in persons with irritable bowel syndrome: Development of a new measure. Digestive Discovery Science. 1998;43:400–11.

Chapter 8
Fibromyalgia

Stella D. Nelms, Kimberly A. Muellers, and Molly A. Warren

Case Vignette

Ms. A is a 62-year-old woman with hypertension, prediabetes, anxiety, depression, and **fibromyalgia** (**FMS**).

Mrs. A.: *I am constantly in pain. Nothing seems to help, and the pain makes it impossible for me to do what I need to do. I am hoping to get some relief.*

Dr. T*: The pain is upsetting and disrupting your life. Tell me what you have tried for this pain.*

Mrs. A: *I saw a rheumatologist 10 years ago who said I have* ***FMS****. He prescribed 60 mg duloxetine in the morning. I don't think it's helping much because I always have pain in my neck and shoulders. The pain is worse if I do housework. I always feel tired. It's hard to stay focused, like I can't think clearly, and my thoughts are cloudy.*

Dr. T: *Although you have an FMS diagnosis, nothing has really helped with pain control. You also have other symptoms that are common in FMS. The mental cloudiness is what we call "brain fog." What have you been told about* ***FMS****?*

Mrs. A: *I know* ***FMS*** *causes pain. I always had anxiety, but these other symptoms started after my son died. Did my son's death cause this?*

S. D. Nelms (✉)
Division of Neuropsychology and Behavioral Health, Department of Rehabilitation Medicine, Emory University School of Medicine, Atlanta, GA, USA
e-mail: stella.d.nelms@emory.edu

K. A. Muellers
Department of Psychology, The New School for Social Research, New York, NY, USA

Department of Psychology, Pace University, New York, NY, USA

M. A. Warren
Direct Primary Care and Acupuncture, Bentleyville, OH, USA

N. Pilipenko, K. M. Desai (eds.), *8 Conditions Primary Care Clinicians Dread to Treat*, https://doi.org/10.1007/978-3-032-12819-5_8

Dr. T: ***FMS** is complex, and we don't know the exact cause.* [Dr. T proceeds to discuss FMS via Message #1.]. *What other questions do you have about FMS?*

Mrs. A: *Can this be cured?*

Dr. T: *While there's no cure for **FMS**, there are strategies we can use to ease your pain and improve your sleep. Would you like me to send you home with more information?*

Mrs. A: Yes, I would like to read more about it.

Dr. T shares resources [see Patient Education Resources] with Mrs. A, and they schedule a follow-up appointment in one month to discuss her treatment goals.

Diagnosis: Brief Description

FMS is characterized by chronic widespread musculoskeletal pain, stiffness, and tenderness, as well as frequent sleep disturbances, cognitive dysfunction, fatigue, and psychiatric symptoms including depression and anxiety [9]. It frequently co-occurs with rheumatologic, psychiatric, and functional somatic conditions [44]. While the etiology of **FMS** is unclear, it likely involves a multifactorial interplay of biological, psychological, and environmental factors, including trauma, chronic stress, repetitive injuries, infections, and obesity [9, 22].

Research suggests that as many as one in twenty people seen in **PC** settings could meet criteria for a **FMS** [30]. Making the diagnosis is often challenging due to the lack of specific biomarkers and overlap with conditions such as lupus, rheumatoid arthritis, diabetes, chronic fatigue syndrome, and multiple sclerosis [23].

Appropriate **FMS** assessment involves reviewing a patient's medical history, performing a physical exam, and using validated symptom screening tools. In clinical practice, **FMS** is most commonly diagnosed using the American College of Rheumatology (ACR) criteria, which require self-reported pain in at least four out of five body regions for three months or longer, with other possible diagnoses excluded [44].

Prevalence, Risk Factors, and Disparities

FMS affects an estimated ten million U.S. adults (3–6% of the population) while its global prevalence ranges from 2% to 4% [29]. These varying estimates reflect ongoing diagnostic challenges and underscore the need for standardized criteria and greater provider education [22].

Overall, several risk factors contribute to **FMS**, including female sex, middle age, genetics, infections, stress, sleep disorders, mental health conditions, and coexisting chronic illnesses [9]. Women aged 30–50 are particularly vulnerable, representing 75–90% of diagnosed cases [24]. Gender bias further complicates diagnosis and treatment: women are more often diagnosed with psychiatric comorbidities, while men with similar symptoms may be overlooked [24].

Disparities in **FMS** extend across both race and socioeconomic status. Black and other non-White patients are underrepresented in research and less likely to receive a formal diagnosis despite comparable or greater symptom burden, especially among Black women [24]. Furthermore, lower socioeconomic status is associated with more severe symptoms, greater functional limitations, and reduced access to care [26]. Collectively, these patterns reveal that **FMS** disproportionately affects women, racial and ethnic minorities, and those with fewer resources, underscoring the need for more equitable research and treatment practices.

Symptom Assessment Tools

Table 8.1 presents three commonly used, validated **FMS** screening tools. The Fibromyalgia Survey Questionnaire (FSQ) is grounded in ACR diagnostic criteria and combines the Widespread Pain Index and Symptom Severity Scale to measure symptom presence, severity, and functional impact [21]. The Fibromyalgia Rapid Screening Tool (FiRST) is designed to quickly identify patients with widespread chronic pain who may warrant further evaluation, making it useful in busy **PC** settings, though it is not diagnostic of **FMS** on its own [33]. Lastly, the Multidimensional Health Assessment Questionnaire (MDHAQ) provides a broader view of patient-reported outcomes such as psychological distress and overall health status [20]. Tool selection depends on clinical purpose: the FSQ is appropriate for confirming diagnosis and assessing severity, while the FiRST for rapid symptom identification, and the MDHAQ for monitoring overall functioning and comorbid concerns.

Non-pharmacological Conceptualization: What to Say to the Patient?

When discussing **FMS** with patients, it is important to frame the discussion within the **biopsychosocial (BPS)** model. Specifically, the **BPS** model proposes that **FMS** symptoms are shaped via an interplay of physical, emotional, and social factors [23]. This model supports a multimodal, individualized approach that integrates education, lifestyle interventions, and psychological support to address the full complexity of the condition and improve outcomes [13]. The following messages illustrate utilization of the **BPS** model in **FMS** care.

Table 8.1 Fibromyalgia assessment screening tools

Screener name	Items #	Rating scale scoring	Cut offs	Assessment timeline	Availability	Psychometric properties	Non-english versions available?
The Fibromyalgia Survey Questionnaire (FSQ) Combines the Widespread Pain Index (WPI) and Symptom Severity Scale (SSS)	WPI: 19 SSS: 6 [45]	WPI: Yes = 1, No = 0 Scale range = 0–19 SSS: Part A 0 = no problem 1 = slight/mild 2 = moderate 3 = severe Part B 0 = no symptoms 1 = few 2 = moderate 3 = many Scale range = 0–12 [45] Total FSQ [17] range = 0–31	WPI: ≥ 7 SSS: ≥5 Diagnosis met if WPI ≥7 and SSS ≥5 = FSQ total score ≥124 [45] Note: the WPI cutoff is ≥7, when paired with SSS ≥ 5	Past 7 days [21, 45]	Open access [21]	WPI Internal consistency [17] = .34 SSS Internal consistency [17] = .83 FSQ Internal consistency [17] = 0.82 Note: All validations involve the entire FSQ.	Spanish (Chile) [1]
Fibromyalgia Rapid Screening Tool (FiRST)	6 [33]	Yes = 1 point, No = 0 [33]	≥5 indicates positive screening [33]	None	Open access [33]	Internal consistency [46] = .96 Cronbach's = 0.79 Sensitivity = 90.5 Specificity = 85.7% [46]	Arabic [2], Spanish [8]
Multi-dimensional Health Assessment Questionnaire (MDHAQ)	10 [34]	0–3 0 = No difficulty, 3 = Unable to do Score 0–10 [34]	Function: 0–30 Pain: 0–10 Global: 0–10 Total range: 0–50 [34]	Past 7 days [34]	Copyrighted [34]	Internal consistency [34] = .84–.94 Function = .85–.95 Pain and Global Health: ~.80–.90	Arabic [14], Chinese [37], Spanish [36]

Message #1: FMS Is a Complex Condition That Requires Holistic Care

FMS is a complex condition with no single known cause. Symptoms such as widespread pain, fatigue, and mood changes can feel overwhelming, but they can be managed by using multiple concurrent strategies. One way to understand **FMS** is to imagine the nervous system as an overly sensitive car alarm. With **FMS**, the alarm can be triggered by even the slightest bump. Triggers such as stress, poor sleep, or **physical activity** can set off this alarm. By recognizing what sets it off, targeted strategies can be used to calm the nervous system and reduce **FMS** symptoms.

Because no single treatment fully addresses these challenges, a holistic approach is essential. This means combining medical care with lifestyle adjustments, psychological support, and self-management strategies.

Why? A wide range of factors can contribute to **FMS** symptom flares. Helping patients to understand this complexity, and the connection between triggers and management strategies, encourages more proactive use of self-management techniques. By framing **FMS** within the **BPS** model, patients are more likely to accept the condition's complexity and remain open to diverse treatment strategies [27].

Message #2: FMS Is Connected to Emotional and Social Factors

Emotional and social factors in **FMS** involve communication between the body and mind. These factors influence symptoms such as pain, fatigue, and sleep disturbances. Addressing anxiety and depression can improve physical functioning and support sustainable treatment. Strong emotional support can improve **FMS** coping. Talking with family, friends, or peers and proactively using strategies to manage stress and mood can enhance overall well-being. Understanding the mind-body connection encourages engagement in strategies that promote emotional resilience, coping skills, and overall well-being.

Why? Psychological distress is common in **FMS** and drives symptom severity and functional impairment. Depression and anxiety can complicate diagnosis and management if left unaddressed [11]. Untreated emotional symptoms can increase pain, worsen fatigue, and disrupt sleep, reducing treatment effectiveness [17, 18, 38]. The relationship is bidirectional: persistent pain can heighten emotional distress, which in turn amplifies physical symptoms through muscle tension and nervous system hyperactivation [10].

Message #3: FMS Can Be Managed, Even If It Cannot Be Cured

FMS is complex and currently has no single cure. Instead, care focuses on management strategies that improve functioning and quality of life. One way to picture this is to imagine building a toolbox, where each tool, such as emotional support, stress management techniques, and lifestyle adjustments, can be used to help manage symptoms when they flare. Over time, using these tools together can calm the “alarm” signals from the nervous system, reducing symptom intensity and frequency while improving resilience and providing a stronger sense of control. Thus, the goal is not to cure **FMS** but to find balance by learning how to manage symptoms so they feel less overwhelming and allow for a better quality of life.

Why? Many patients with **FMS** often struggle with feelings of hopelessness and frustration when they are told there is no cure [6]. Reframing treatment around achievable, evidence-based strategies can restore hope and promote active coping. For example, support groups can provide emotional validation, reduce isolation, and offer opportunies to share practical coping strategies [35] (see Resources for support groups). Similarly, community-based interventions that include pain education, physical exercise, and peer support have been shown to significantly improve functioning, satisfaction with care, pain beliefs, and depressive symptoms [40]. Providing the rationale behind this approach helps patients understand the purpose of their treatment plan, increases adherence, and counters stigma by reinforcing that **FMS** is a legitimate clinical condition [13].

Case Vignette—Continued

Mrs. A returns for her one-month follow-up appointment.

Mrs. A*: Reading the handouts on **FMS** has helped me understand my symptoms better. But I’m still worried I won’t get relief from all my pain. The duloxetine hasn’t helped. What else can I do?*

Dr. T: *Gentle exercise can make a real difference in **FMS** pain. What kind of movement are you doing now?*

Mrs. A: *I clean my house, but otherwise, I don’t exercise. Sometimes I feel like it makes my pain worse.*

Dr. T: *That’s a common concern. The key is choosing gentle, low-impact activities—like tai chi or swimming—which can reduce pain without overloading your body. If we push too hard, pain can flare. What kinds of movement have you enjoyed in the past?*

Mrs. A: *I used to go to swimming classes for seniors at the community center. I liked it because it was fun, and I had friends there.*

Dr. T: *Let the instructor know that you may want to take breaks during class.* Dr. T proceeds to discuss activity **pacing** in **FMS** [see Teach activity modification: **Pacing**].

Mrs. A: *Okay, I'll try to schedule a few breaks in my class. How often should I go?*
Dr. T: *Let's set a realistic goal together. How many times a week do you think you could go to swimming classes between now and then?*
Mrs. A: *I think I could go on Mondays and Fridays.*
Dr. T: *Perfect. Twice a week is a great starting point. Before we wrap up, let's rate your pain. On a scale of 1–10—where 10 is the worst pain imaginable—how would you rate your pain on most days?*
Mrs. A: *Most days it's about a 7, mostly in my neck and shoulders. Today it's 8. So, I'll plan to go twice a week for the next four weeks?*
Dr. T: *Exactly. Can you come back to see me in about four weeks, and we'll review your pain and make adjustments if needed?*
Mrs. A: *Sure. I can do that.*

Non-pharmacological Treatment Options: What Can Be Done?

Non-pharmacological interventions are vital to **FMS** management and can be effectively integrated into **PC**. Three core strategies include supporting regular **physical activity**, teaching **pacing**, and promoting **symptom tracking**.

1. **Support Regular Physical Activity Engagement**

Patients who are deconditioned or new to exercise can benefit from beginning with low-impact activities such as walking, swimming, yoga, or gentle stretching. It is important to emphasize a "start low, go slow" approach to help patients recognize their physical limits and prevent pain flares. For example, the American College of Sports Medicine recommends engaging in 10–20 min of low-impact exercise for a duration of 2–3 days per week, as well as incorporating approximately 30 minutes of strength-training exercises 2–3 times per week [7].

Physicians can promote effective activity engagement by helping patients set Specific, Measurable, Achievable, Relevant, and Time-bound (SMART) goals for **physical activity** [43]. For example, instead of a vague goal "exercise more," a SMART goal might be, "Walk for 10 minutes, three times a week for the next two weeks." Physicians should collaborate with patients to set realistic goals, monitor progress, and gradually increase activity levels.

Why? Physical activity is one of the most evidence-supported interventions for managing **FMS** [29]. Regular aerobic exercise, as well as strength and flexibility training, can reduce pain, improve mobility, and decrease inflammation [44].

2. **Teach Activity Modification: Pacing**

Pacing strategies can help prevent both overexertion and activity avoidance, common contributors to symptom flare-ups in **FMS** [3]. Effective **pacing** involves:

- Alternating activity and rest: Encourage patients to schedule rest breaks before exhaustion sets in. For example, after 15 minutes of **physical activity,** take a five-minute break before resuming.
- Breaking tasks into smaller steps: For example, before cleaning the entire house at once, clean one room, rest, and then resume later.
- Identifying symptom triggers: Help patients reflect on activities that consistently worsen pain or fatigue, and adjust the intensity, duration, or frequency accordingly. For example, if high-impact exercise triggers symptom flares, substitute with low-impact activity such as walking or yoga.

Why? Both overactivity and inactivity can worsen pain, fatigue, and functional limitations [3]. **Pacing** strategies help patients gradually build endurance without exacerbating symptoms and support long-term engagement in **physical activity**. Consistent **physical activity** can improve pain, mood, sleep, and overall function in individuals with **FMS** [7].

3. **Encourage Self-Monitoring/Symptom Tracking**
   Use of diaries or apps to record pain, fatigue, and **physical activity** helps patients identify symptom triggers and patterns, adjust behaviors, and communicate more effectively with healthcare providers (see Resources for tracking tools).
   Why? This strategy empowers patients to take control of their symptoms while providing healthcare providers accurate data on symptom fluctuations [19]. For example, a randomized controlled trial (RCT) of 40 participants using a digital app and paper-and-pencil tracking showed moderate improvement of symptom severity from baseline [47].

Psychotherapy Effectiveness

Considerable evidence supports psychological therapies, specifically cognitive behavioral therapy (CBT) and acceptance and commitment therapy (ACT), as central components of effective **FMS** management [5, 39]. These interventions target the cognitive, emotional, and behavioral aspects of **FMS** and enhance resilience, improve functioning and mood, and reduce the impact of symptoms on daily life [5]. CBT's flexibility makes it particularly well suited to **PC**, as it can be delivered in brief sessions [4].

Brief CBT modules emphasizing psychoeducation, goal setting, **pacing**, and relaxation techniques have been linked to the greatest treatment gains [4]. Specifically, moderate treatment effects (Cohen's $d = 0.65$) for measures of pain intensity and functional limitations were found, indicating that these interventions had a meaningful impact on patient outcomes. Meta-analyses and recent trials report moderate effects of CBT in reducing depression and anxiety [5, 12] and small-to-moderate improvements in pain and health-related quality of life [5]. Importantly, CBT can reduce pain interference by addressing pain catastrophizing and maladaptive thought patterns.

Integrative Medicine Interventions and Techniques

Mind-body interventions—including **tai chi**, **acupuncture**, **mindfulness**, and **massage**—are commonly used to help alleviate **FMS** symptoms such as pain, fatigue, anxiety, and depression [28]. The following sections summarize the evidence for each approach.

Acupuncture

Acupuncture may reduce pain and stiffness in **FMS**, likely through the release of neurotransmitters such as endorphins and serotonin [31]. A meta-analysis of 12 RCTs found significant pain reduction, with an average improvement of 1 point on the pain Visual Analogue Scale (VAS). Pain improvement was sustained for 6 months, with a 2-point greater reduction in VAS scores compared with conventional medications. Significant improvements in quality of life were also observed on the Fibromyalgia Impact Questionnaire (FIQ), with a mean improvement of 16.72 points [48].

Massage and Manual Therapy

Myofascial release (MFR) is a specialized manual therapy technique involving gentle, sustained pressure applied to fascial tissue. MFR is performed by a physical therapist, occupational therapist, or **massage** therapist with specialty training. Meta-analytic data indicate that MFR (one weekly session for 20 weeks) led to significant reductions in pain with a mean reduction of 0.81 points on the VAS, as well as improvements in anxiety, depression, and sleep [41].

Tai Chi

Tai chi, a practice involving slow, gentle movements and postures, has been shown to improve psychological well-being and functional ability in **FMS** [28]. Participating in **tai chi** for 24 weeks was associated with significantly greater pain reduction compared with aerobic exercise. Although both groups reported pain improvement, **tai chi** produced significantly greater benefits, with a mean difference of 16.2 points in total FIQ scores. **Tai chi** also led to significant improvements in anxiety (−1.2 points), self-efficacy (+1.0 point), and coping strategies (+2.6 points) [42]. Physicians may encourage patients to explore **tai chi** through in-person classes or instructional videos available online (see Resources).

Mindfulness

Mindfulness-based stress reduction (MBSR) is a structured program that incorporates meditation, gentle yoga, and relaxation techniques to reduce pain, fatigue, and mood disturbances. In a RCT of 225 patients with **FMS**, participants were assigned to MBSR plus treatment as usual, treatment as usual alone, or a multicomponent **FMS** program without MBSR. MBSR combined with usual care was superior to the comparison groups, with a number needed to treat of four to achieve a 20% reduction in FIQR scores [32]. Physicians may also consider directing patients to free online MBSR programs (see Resources).

Supplements

Vitamin D supplementation may be beneficial for patients with **FMS** and comorbid vitamin D deficiency. In a 2023 cross-sectional clinical study, 180 women with **FMS** and vitamin D deficiency received 50,000 IU of oral vitamin D_3 weekly for 12 weeks. Improvements were observed in pain, with a 2.55-point reduction on the VAS, and in quality of life, with a mean improvement of 13.81 points on the FIQ [15]. Physicians should test 25-OH vitamin D levels in patients with **FMS** and initiate treatment if deficiency is present.

Clinical Pearls

- Frame **FMS** within the **BPS** model. Explain that symptoms can arise from an interaction of physical, emotional, and social factors.
- Promote a holistic and multimodal management approach. Emphasize that no single treatment is sufficient; combining medical care, lifestyle adjustments, psychological support, and self-management strategies improves outcomes.
- Discuss setting realistic goals and expectations. Reinforce that focus is on symptom management and improved functioning rather than cure.
- Encourage practical strategies. Support incorporating **physical activity**, **pacing**, and **symptom tracking**, and explaining the rationale behind these interventions to improve adherence.

Frequently Asked Questions

Question 1: *How do you diagnose **FMS**?*
Answer: There's no single test. **FMS** is diagnosed based on your symptoms, screening tools, and ruling out other conditions with lab tests.

Question 2: *What options do I have other than medication?*

Answer: Non-medication options include gentle exercise (e.g., walking, **tai chi**), physical therapy, stress-reduction techniques like CBT or **mindfulness**, and complementary therapies such as **acupuncture** or manual **massage** therapy.

Question 3: *Won't exercise make my symptoms/pain worse?*

Answer: Pain during exercise is common, but starting slowly with low-impact, enjoyable activities—like walking, swimming, or **tai chi**, and gradually increasing intensity can help reduce pain and improve function.

Question 4: *How could psychotherapy make a difference in managing my symptoms?*

Answer: Evidence-based therapies like CBT can reduce stress, change unhelpful thoughts, and support healthy behaviors, including regular **physical activity**, improved sleep, and effective coping strategies for managing **FMS** symptoms.

Resources

Source	Description	Link
Patient education resources		
Mayo Clinic	Educational information on symptoms, causes, diagnosis, treatment options, and clinical trials. Available in Spanish text	https://www.mayoclinic.org/diseases-conditions/fibromyalgia/symptoms-causes/syc-20354780
American College of Rheumatology (ACR)	Brief printable fact sheet on FMS signs/symptoms and treatment options	https://rheumatology.org/patients/fibromyalgia
American College of Rheumatology (ACR)	Brief printable fact sheet on FMS signs/symptoms and treatment options in Spanish text	https://rheumatology.org/patients/fibromialgia
Tracking resources		
Bearable	Free app that offers symptom tracking, mood, sleep, medication logs, and daily reminders	https://bearable.app/
Guava	Free app that offers symptom tracking, mood and medication logs, and a "heat map" view of symptom locations	https://guavahealth.com/
MBSR and therapy resources		
Curable	Free interactive app that provides pain education, CBT, and mindfulness exercises	https://www.curablehealth.com/
Stanza	Prescription based app that delivers a 12-week self-Guided ACT program	https://swingtherapeutics.com/stanza/
Palouse Mindfulness	Free online 8-week MBSR course that offers a certificate of completion	https://palousemindfulness.com/index.html

(continued)

Source	Description	Link
Bilingual Center for Mindfulness	Offers free guided meditations and mindfulness exercises in Spanish	https://bilingualmindfulness.com/
MyFibroTeam	Offers information on support groups	https://www.myfibroteam.com/
Tai Chi		
Tai Chi Instructional Video	Beginners instructional video	https://www.youtube.com/watch?v=bcpelNJTDbY

Case Vignette—Conclusion

Mrs. A returns four weeks later for a follow-up appointment.

Dr. T: *At our last visit, we set a goal of going swimming twice a week at your community center. How did this go for you?*

Mrs. A: *There was one week that I only went once, but otherwise, I went twice per week. It was helpful that I met a few friends through the class, so I look forward to going.*

Dr. T: *Did you notice any changes to your pain in connection with swimming? Can you rate your pain for me today?*

Mrs. A: *My pain in my neck and shoulders has been around 3 or 4 for the past two weeks, and today it is a 4.*

Dr. T: *You mentioned at our last visit that your pain was usually a 7 or 8, is this correct?*

Mrs. A: *Yes, my pain is a little better. However, I still feel anxious and sad most days.*

Dr. T: *You told me before that your symptoms were worse after your son's death.* ***FMS*** *is complex. It can cause more anxiety and depression, and our mood can worsen other* ***FMS*** *symptoms. We have a few options to support your mood. Would you be interested in learning more about speaking with a trained therapist, or exploring* ***mindfulness*** *activities you can do at home on your own?*

Mrs. A: *I'm nervous to talk to someone. I think I would rather do something on my own. What is* ***mindfulness****?*

Dr. T: ***Mindfulness*** *is the practice of focusing on the present moment in a calm, non-judgmental way to reduce stress. It often involves noticing sensations within our bodies. Practicing* ***mindfulness*** *can help reduce symptoms of anxiety. Can I share free online resources with you for activities you can do at home?*

Mrs. A: *Sure, I would like to try this.*

Dr. T proceeds to share the Palouse **Mindfulness** (see Resources) and schedules a three-month follow-up.

References

1. Aguirre Cárdenas C, Oñederra MC, Esparza Benavente C, Durán J, González Tugas M, Gómez-Pérez L. Psychometric properties of the Fibromyalgia Survey Questionnaire in Chilean women with fibromyalgia. J Clin Rheumatol. 2021;27(6S):S284–93. https://doi.org/10.1097/RHU.0000000000001547.
2. Alshubaili A, Al-Badri F, Al-Zoubi S. Validation of the Arabic version of the Fibromyalgia Rapid Screening Tool (FiRST) among patients with chronic pain. J Pain Res. 2021;14:3297–305. https://doi.org/10.2147/JPR.S317250.
3. Barakou I, Hackett KL, Finch T, Hettinga FJ. Self-regulation of effort for a better health-related quality of life: a multidimensional activity pacing model for chronic pain and fatigue management. Ann Med. 2023;55(2):2270688. https://doi.org/10.1080/07853890.2023.2270688.
4. Beehler GP, Murphy JL, King PR, Dollar KM, Kearney LK, Haslam A, Wade M, Goldstein WR. Brief cognitive behavioral therapy for chronic pain: results from a clinical demonstration project in primary care behavioral health. Clin J Pain. 2019;35(10):809–17. https://doi.org/10.1097/AJP.0000000000000747.
5. Bernardy K, Klose P, Welsch P, Häuser W. Efficacy, acceptability and safety of cognitive behavioural therapies in fibromyalgia syndrome - a systematic review and meta-analysis of randomized controlled trials. Eur J Pain. 2018;22(2):242–60. https://doi.org/10.1002/ejp.1121.
6. Briones-Vozmediano E, Vives-Cases C, Ronda-Pérez E, Gil-González D. Patients' and professionals' views on managing fibromyalgia. Pain Res Manag. 2013;18(1):19–24. https://doi.org/10.1155/2013/742510.
7. Busch AJ, Webber SC, Brachaniec M, Bidonde J, Bello-Haas VD, Danyliw AD, Overend TJ, Richards RS, Sawant A, Schachter CL. Exercise therapy for fibromyalgia. Curr Pain Headache Rep. 2011;15(5):358–67. https://doi.org/10.1007/s11916-011-0214-2.
8. Casanueva B, Belenguer R, Moreno-Muelas JV, Urtiaga J, Urtiaga B, Hernández JL, Pina T, González-Gay MA. Validation of the Spanish version of the Fibromyalgia Rapid Screening Tool to detect fibromyalgia in primary care health centres. Clin Exp Rheumatol. 2016;34(2, Suppl. 96):S125–8.
9. Centers for Disease Control and Prevention. Fibromyalgia. 2024. https://www.cdc.gov/arthritis/fibromyalgia/.
10. Chang M-H, Hsu J-W, Huang K-L, Su T-P, Bai Y-M, Li C-T, Yang AC, Chang W-H, Chen T-J, Tsai S-J, Chen M-H. Bidirectional association between depression and fibromyalgia syndrome: a nationwide longitudinal study. J Pain. 2015;16(9):873–80. https://doi.org/10.1016/j.jpain.2015.05.002.
11. Clauw DJ. Fibromyalgia: A clinical review. JAMA. 2014;311(15):1547–55. https://doi.org/10.1001/jama.2014.3266.
12. Cojocaru CM, Popa CO, Schenk A, Suciu BA, Szasz S. Cognitive-behavioral therapy and acceptance and commitment therapy for anxiety and depression in patients with fibromyalgia: a systematic review and meta-analysis. Med Pharm Rep. 2024;97(1):26–34. https://doi.org/10.15386/mpr-2661.
13. Duhn PH, Wæhrens EE, Pedersen MB, Nielsen SM, Locht H, Bliddal H, Christensen R, Amris K. Effectiveness of patient education as a stand-alone intervention for patients with chronic widespread pain and fibromyalgia: a systematic review and meta-analysis of randomized trials. Scand J Rheumatol. 2023;52(6):654–63. https://doi.org/10.1080/03009742.2023.2192450.
14. El Miedany Y, El Gaafary M, Youssef SS, Ahmed I. Validity of the developed Arabic Multidimensional Health Assessment Questionnaire for use in standard clinical care of patients with rheumatic diseases. Int J Rheum Dis. 2008;11(3):246–55. https://doi.org/10.1111/j.1756-185X.2008.00366.x.
15. Ersoy S, Kesiktas FN, Sirin B, Bugdayci D, Paker N. The effect of vitamin D treatment on quality of life in patients with fibromyalgia. Ir J Med Sci. 2024;193(2):1111–6. https://doi.org/10.1007/s11845-023-03521-4.

16. Fitzcharles M-A, Ste-Marie PA, Panopalis P, Menard J, Shir Y, Wolfe F. The 2010 American College of Rheumatology fibromyalgia survey diagnostic criteria and symptom severity scale is a valid and reliable tool in a French speaking fibromyalgia cohort. BMC Musculoskelet Disord. 2012;13:179. https://doi.org/10.1186/1471-2474-13-179.
17. Gálvez-Sánchez CM, de la Coba P, Duschek S, Reyes del Paso GA. Reliability, factor structure and predictive validity of the Widespread Pain Index and Symptom Severity scales of the 2010 American College of Rheumatology criteria of fibromyalgia. J Clin Med. 2020;9(8):2460. https://doi.org/10.3390/jcm9082460.
18. Gálvez-Sánchez CM, Montoro CI, Duschek S, Reyes del Paso GA. Depression and trait-anxiety mediate the influence of clinical pain on health-related quality of life in fibromyalgia. J Affect Disord. 2020b;265:486–95. https://doi.org/10.1016/j.jad.2020.01.129.
19. Garcia-Palacios A, Herrero R, Belmonte MA, Castilla D, Guixeres J, Molinari G, Baños RM. Ecological momentary assessment for chronic pain in fibromyalgia using a smartphone: a randomized crossover study. Eur J Pain. 2014;18(6):862–72. https://doi.org/10.1002/j.1532-2149.2013.00425.x.
20. Gibson KA, Castrejon I, Descallar J, Pincus T. Fibromyalgia assessment screening tool: clues to fibromyalgia on a Multidimensional Health Assessment Questionnaire for routine care. J Rheumatol. 2020;47(5):761–9. https://doi.org/10.3899/jrheum.190277.
21. Häuser W, Jung E, Erbslöh-Möller B, Gesmann M, Kühn-Becker H, Petermann F, Langhorst J, Weiss T, Winkelmann A, Wolfe F. Validation of the Fibromyalgia Survey Questionnaire within a cross-sectional survey. PLoS One. 2012;7(5):e37504. https://doi.org/10.1371/journal.pone.0037504.
22. Häuser W, Ablin J, Fitzcharles MA, Littlejohn G, Luciano JV, Usui C, Walitt B. Fibromyalgia. Nat Rev Dis Primers. 2015;1:15022. https://doi.org/10.1038/nrdp.2015.22.
23. Häuser W, Sarzi-Puttini P, Fitzcharles MA. Fibromyalgia syndrome: Under-, over- and misdiagnosis. Clin Exp Rheumatol. 2019;37(Suppl. 116):90–7.
24. Jacobs M, Crall E, Menzies V. Fibromyalgia syndrome among men and women: symptom identification, diagnosis, and concurrence in a nationally representative sample. Open Rheumatol J. 2024;19. https://doi.org/10.2174/0118743129356140241217040050.
25. Lee J, Lazaridou A, Paschali M, Loggia ML, Berry MP, Ellingsen DM, Isenburg K, Anzolin A, Grahl A, Wasan AD, Napadow V, Edwards RR. A randomized controlled neuroimaging trial of cognitive behavioral therapy for fibromyalgia pain. Arthritis Rheumatol. 2024;76(1):130–40. https://doi.org/10.1002/art.42672.
26. Mathkhor AJ, Atwan AH. Fibromyalgia syndrome and its allied clinical features are associated with low socioeconomic status. Int J Clin Rheumtol. 2022;17(11):163–8.
27. Mengshoel AM, Skarbø Å, Hasselknippe E, Petterson T, Brandsar NL, Askmann E, Ildstad R, Løseth L, Sallinen MH. Enabling personal recovery from fibromyalgia—theoretical rationale, content and meaning of a person-centred, recovery-oriented programme. BMC Health Serv Res. 2021;21(1):339. https://doi.org/10.1186/s12913-021-06295-6.
28. National Center for Complementary and Integrative Health. Mind and body practices for fibromyalgia: what the science says. 2021. https://www.nccih.nih.gov/health/providers/digest/mind-and-body-practices-for-fibromyalgia-science.
29. National Fibromyalgia Association. All about fibromyalgia. 2025. https://www.fmaware.org/fibromyalgia/.
30. National Institute of Arthritis and Musculoskeletal and Skin Diseases. (n.d.). Fibromyalgia. U.S. Department of Health and Human Services, National Institutes of Health. https://www.niams.nih.gov/health-topics/fibromyalgia.
31. Patil S, Sen S, Bral M, Reddy S, Bradley KK, Cornett EM, Fox CJ, Kaye AD. The role of acupuncture in pain management. Curr Pain Headache Rep. 2016;20(4):22. https://doi.org/10.1007/s11916-016-0552-1.
32. Pérez-Aranda A, Feliu-Soler A, Montero-Marín J, García-Campayo J, Andrés-Rodríguez L, Borràs X, Rozadilla-Sacanell A, Peñarrubia-Maria MT, Angarita-Osorio N, McCracken LM, Luciano JV. A randomized controlled efficacy trial of mindfulness-based stress reduction com-

pared with an active control group and usual care for fibromyalgia: the EUDAIMON study. Pain. 2019;160(11):2508–23. https://doi.org/10.1097/j.pain.0000000000001655.

33. Perrot S, Bouhassira D, Fermanian J. Development and validation of the Fibromyalgia Rapid Screening Tool (FiRST). Pain. 2010;150(2):250–6. https://doi.org/10.1016/j.pain.2010.03.034.
34. Pincus T, Swearingen C, Wolfe F. A multidimensional Health Assessment Questionnaire (MDHAQ) for all rheumatic diseases to complete at all visits in standard clinical care. Arthritis Rheum. 2005;52(10):3184–91. https://doi.org/10.1002/art.21214.
35. Reig-Garcia G, Bosch-Farré C, Suñer-Soler R, Juvinyà-Canal D, Pla-Vila N, Noell-Boix R, Boix-Roqueta E, Mantas-Jiménez S. The impact of a peer social support network from the perspective of women with fibromyalgia: a qualitative study. Int J Environ Res Public Health. 2021;18(23):12801. https://doi.org/10.3390/ijerph182312801.
36. RWS Life Sciences. MDHAQ-RAPID3 available translations languages. n.d. https://life-sciences.rws.com/mdhaq-rapid3/translations/available-translations.
37. Song Y, Zhu L-A, Wang S-L, Leng L, Bucala R, Lu L-J. Multi-dimensional health assessment questionnaire in China: reliability, validity, and clinical value in patients with rheumatoid arthritis. PLoS One. 2014;9(5):e97952. https://doi.org/10.1371/journal.pone.0097952.
38. Taylor S, Furness P, Ashe S, Haywood-Small S, Lawson K. Comorbid conditions, mental health and cognitive functions in adults with fibromyalgia. West J Nurs Res. 2020;43(2):115–22. https://doi.org/10.1177/0193945920937429.
39. Thieme K, Mathys M, Turk DC. Evidence-based guidelines on the treatment of fibromyalgia patients: are they consistent and if not, why not? Have effective psychological treatments been overlooked? J Pain. 2017;18(7):747–56.
40. Turcotte K, Oelke ND, Whitaker G, Holtzman S, O'Connor B, Pearson N, Teo M. Multidisciplinary community-based group intervention for fibromyalgia: a pilot randomized controlled trial. Rheumatol Int. 2023;43(12):2201–10. https://doi.org/10.1007/s00296-023-05403-5.
41. Ughreja RA, Venkatesan P, Balebail Gopalakrishna D, Singh YP. Effectiveness of myofascial release on pain, sleep, and quality of life in patients with fibromyalgia syndrome: a systematic review. Complement Ther Clin Pract. 2021;45:101477. https://doi.org/10.1016/j.ctcp.2021.101477.
42. Wang C, Schmid CH, Fielding RA, Harvey WF, Reid KF, Price LL, Driban JB, Kalish R, Rones R, McAlindon T. Effect of tai chi versus aerobic exercise for fibromyalgia: comparative effectiveness randomized controlled trial. BMJ. 2018;360:k851. https://doi.org/10.1136/bmj.k851.
43. White ND, Bautista V, Lenz T, Cosimano A. Using the SMART-EST goals in lifestyle medicine prescription. Am J Lifestyle Med. 2020;14(3):271–3. https://doi.org/10.1177/1559827620905775.
44. Winslow BT, Vandal C, Dang L. Fibromyalgia: diagnosis and management. Am Fam Physician. 2023;107(2):137–44.
45. Wolfe F, Clauw DJ, Fitzcharles MA, Goldenberg DL, Katz RS, Mease P, Russell AS, Russell IJ, Winfield JB, Yunus MB. The American College of Rheumatology preliminary diagnostic criteria for fibromyalgia and measurement of symptom severity. Arthritis Care Res. 2010;62(5):600–10. https://doi.org/10.1002/acr.20140.
46. Wroński J, Rozenek H, Włodarczyk D. Validation of the Fibromyalgia Rapid Screening Tool in patients with axial spondyloarthritis: polish version adaptation and value in clinical practice. Pol Arch Intern Med. 2024;134(7–8):16753. https://doi.org/10.20452/pamw.16753.
47. Yuan SLK, Couto LA, Marques AP. Effects of a six-week mobile app versus paper book intervention on quality of life, symptoms, and self-care in patients with fibromyalgia: a randomized parallel trial. Braz J Phys Ther. 2021;25(4):428–36. https://doi.org/10.1016/j.bjpt.2020.10.003.
48. Zhang XC, Chen H, Xu WT, Song YY, Gu YH, Ni GX. Acupuncture therapy for fibromyalgia: a systematic review and meta-analysis of randomized controlled trials. J Pain Res. 2019;12:527–42. https://doi.org/10.2147/JPR.S186227.

Chapter 9
Headache

Stella D. Nelms, Kimberly A. Muellers, and Sharon Chacko

Case Vignette

Ms. A is a 40-year-old woman who presents to her primary care (PC) provider with complaints of long-standing headaches. Additionally, she has a history of insomnia and gestational hypertension.

Ms. A: *My headaches have been getting worse lately. I used to only get them around my period or when I was really stressed, but now I'm having them at least once a week.*

Dr. L: *Let's talk more about what you're experiencing and see how I can help. I hear that the frequency of your headaches has increased and you are concerned. How have you been managing the headaches?*

Ms. A: *Sometimes I take ibuprofen. It helps occasionally, but other times it feels like I take it too late—by then it's already turned into a migraine with nausea, and I just have to lie down in a dark, quiet room until it passes.*

Dr. L: *So sometimes the ibuprofen helps, but other times the headache worsens, maybe because you take the medication too late.*

Ms. A: *Yes, exactly!*

S. D. Nelms (✉)
Division of Neuropsychology and Behavioral Health, Department of Rehabilitation Medicine, Emory University School of Medicine, Atlanta, GA, USA
e-mail: stella.d.nelms@emory.edu

K. A. Muellers
Department of Psychology, The New School for Social Research, New York, NY, USA

Department of Psychology, Pace University, New York, NY, USA

S. Chacko
Center for Family and Community Medicine, Department of Medicine, NewYork-Presbyterian Hospital/Columbia University Irving Medical Center, New York, NY, USA

N. Pilipenko, K. M. Desai (eds.), *8 Conditions Primary Care Clinicians Dread to Treat*, https://doi.org/10.1007/978-3-032-12819-5_9

Dr. L: *Last time we spoke about your headaches, you mentioned that your headaches don't come along with any other symptoms like fever, eye pain, blurry vision, or muscle weakness. They aren't triggered by positional changes or things like coughing or exercise. The pattern of your headaches is the same as usual, and you've never had cancer. I just wanted to confirm all of this.*

Ms. A: *Yes, that's all correct.*

Dr. L: *Have you ever kept a diary of your headaches?*

Ms. A: *This seems like a lot of work. What's the point of doing all of this? I just told you all about my headaches.*

Dr. L: *You have a lot of insight into your headaches and gave me a lot of information about your symptoms. What are your goals regarding your headaches?*

Ms. A: *I want to have fewer headaches.*

Dr. L: *Headaches can be tricky to manage because various things can trigger them.* ***Tracking*** *is the best way to identify your specific triggers, and it can help us make the best treatment plan to reach your goal and have fewer days with headaches. Do you think you can keep the log over the next month until our next appointment?* (see Resources for options for symptom **tracking** and headache diaries).

Ms. A: *If you think it will help us get to the bottom of my headaches and help me have more headache-free days, then I will.*

Diagnosis: Brief Description

The International Classification of **Headache Disorders,** 3rd Edition [15] categorizes **headache disorders (HDs)** into three groups: primary headaches (PHs), secondary headaches (SHs), and painful cranial neuropathies, other facial pains, and other headaches (CNFPs). PHs are diagnosed based on symptom patterns and the exclusion of secondary causes [19] and include **tension-type headaches (TTH)**, **migraine**, and **cluster headache**. SHs result from underlying conditions such as trauma, infection, or vascular abnormalities and often require further diagnostic evaluation with imaging or laboratory tests. CNFPs stem from cranial nerve dysfunction and typically require specialized assessment [7, 15]. For detailed diagnostic criteria and classification guidelines across all headache types, physicians can consult the ICHD-3.

This chapter focuses on PHs, as these are the most prevalent. The most common presentations include:

- ***Tension-Type Headache (TTH)***: Typically bilateral with a pressing or tightening quality. The pain is mild to moderate, not aggravated by physical activity, and usually not associated with nausea or vomiting.
- ***Migraine:*** Often unilateral and pulsating, **migraines** are moderate to severe in intensity and worsen with activity. These are commonly accompanied by nausea, vomiting, photophobia, and phonophobia. A subset of patients experience aura, consisting of transient visual, sensory, or speech disturbances.

- ***Cluster Headache***: Severe, unilateral orbital or temporal pain that occurs in cyclical patterns (e.g., daily for several weeks). Episodes are brief but intense and are often accompanied by autonomic symptoms such as tearing, nasal congestion, or ptosis [15].

Diagnosing **HDs** begins with a thorough patient history and physical examination. A focused history includes symptom onset, frequency, duration, intensity, and location of pain, as well as associated symptoms (e.g., nausea, photophobia, phonophobia, aura) and potential triggers such as stress, hormonal changes, or specific foods [17]. Imaging is typically reserved for patients presenting with "red flag" features, including signs of infection, trauma, or neurologic deficits [39].

Prevalence, Risk Factors, and Disparities

PHs vary in prevalence, risk profiles, and impact across populations. Specifically, **TTH** affects approximately 38% of adults worldwide each year. Despite its high prevalence, **TTH** is frequently underreported. It is more common in women, with a female-to-male ratio of approximately 1.5:1 [39]. **Migraine** affects approximately 12% of adults in the United States (U.S.), with women being nearly three times more likely to experience **migraines** than men [5]. Finally, **cluster headaches**, while far less common, affect about 0.1% of the U.S. population and occur approximately three times more often in men than in women [16].

Risk factors differ among headache types. For **TTH**, these include younger age, insomnia, psychological stress, and musculoskeletal tension. **Migraine** risk is associated with genetic predisposition, psychiatric comorbidities (e.g., depression, anxiety), hormonal fluctuations, and dietary triggers (e.g., alcohol and processed foods). **Cluster headaches** are linked to family history and tobacco exposure [8].

Significant disparities exist in the diagnosis and management of **HDs** based on race/ethnicity, socioeconomic status, and access to care [18]. Black and Hispanic patients are 25–50% less likely to receive a **migraine** diagnosis compared with White patients, despite reporting similar or greater symptom burden [5]. Additionally, historical medical mistrust among African Americans contributes to lower utilization of healthcare services for headache treatment, resulting in lower rates of diagnosis and prescription of appropriate medications [11].

Symptom Assessment Tools

Symptom assessment tools can support diagnosis, measure severity, and monitor the impact of **HDs** on daily functioning. Table 9.1 highlights three commonly used instruments that share several features: all are validated, brief, self-administered questionnaires designed to improve clinical decision-making in both primary and

Table 9.1 Headache disorder screening tools

Screener name	Items #	Rating scale scoring	Cut offs	Assessment timeline	Availability	Psychometric properties	Non-english versions available?
ID Migraine™	3 [24]	Yes/No [24] Yes = 1 point No = 0 points Total possible: 0–3	2 or more "Yes" responses	0–90 days [24]	Open Access [24]	Sensitivity = 81% Specificity = 75% Positive predictive value = 93% in PC settings [24]	Arabic [1], Chinese [40], Spanish [33]
Headache Impact Test (HIT-6™)	6 [30]	5-point likert [30] 36 (lowest impact) to 78 (highest impact) [30]	≥56: Substantial impact (suggestive of migraine) ≥60: Severe impact ≤49: Little/no impact ≥6-point decrease = Clinically meaningful improvement	Past few weeks to 1 month [30]	Copyrighted [30]	Internal consistency = .82–.90 Test-retest reliability = .77–.80 [30]	Arabic [14]
Migraine Disability Assessment (MIDAS)	7 [36]	5 disability-related items 2 unscored items for headache frequency & pain intensity (0–10) Counts of days Sum of items 1–5 [36]	Disability grade cutoffs [36] 0–5: Little or no disability (Grade I) 6–10: Mild (Grade II) 11–20: Moderate (Grade III) 1+: Severe (Grade IV)	0–90 days [36]	Open access [35]	Internal consistency = .83 Test-retest reliability = .81–.90 [35]	Arabic [26], Spanish [25, 32]

specialty care settings. Specifically, the ID **Migraine**™ can efficiently assess **migraine** symptoms, including nausea, photophobia, and activity limitation in **PC** [24]. The **Migraine** Disability Assessment (MIDAS) evaluates three-month prevalence of **migraine**-related disability and functional limitations and provides guidance for treatment planning [36]. The Headache Impact Test (HIT-6™) assesses the broader impact of headaches on quality of life, including pain severity, emotional distress, and daily functioning [30]. The ID **Migraine**™ functions primarily as a diagnostic screener, whereas the MIDAS and HIT-6™ are more useful for monitoring severity and functional impact over time.

Non-pharmacological Conceptualization: What to Say to the Patient?

While medications can help reduce headache frequency and/or severity, they are not universally effective and may cause side effects or medication overuse [22]. Therefore, non-pharmacological strategies are essential for both prevention and management. The **biopsychosocial (BPS)** approach provides a useful framework for these strategies by emphasizing that headaches are influenced by a confluence of biological mechanisms, stress, lifestyle behaviors, and thought patterns [20]. The **BPS** approach facilitates personalized interventions and may reduce reliance on medication [4].

Message #1: Multiple Factors Contribute to Headaches

HDs can have different causes. When creating a treatment plan, it's important to look at all possible factors—including biological, behavioral, and psychosocial—that may play a role. If triggers are managed, headaches can be prevented or become less frequent. This in turn can reduce the need for medication and improve quality of life.

Why? Engaging patients in collaborative discussions about factors which lead to headaches fosters a shared understanding of symptoms and encourages partnership in care [20]. Framing education as a partnership can increase patient engagement, validate experiences, enhance self-efficacy, and support long-term self-management [12].

Message #2: A Multimodal Treatment Plan Is Key

The best results in managing headaches usually come from a mix of strategies that are tailored to the individual patient. These might include dietary modifications, regular physical activity, adequate sleep, and stress management, along with any prescribed medications.

Why? A personalized, multimodal plan offers greater flexibility, reduces reliance on medication, and lowers the risk of adverse effects or overuse. Evidence suggests that integrating pharmacological and **non-pharmacological** strategies such as **biofeedback**, relaxation techniques, and lifestyle modifications, leads to more sustainable improvements in headache management [22]. Benefits include sustained reductions in headache frequency and severity, as well as improved patient self-efficacy in managing symptoms.

Message #3: Realistic Expectations Are Important

HDs are typically chronic or recurrent, and treatment rarely eliminates them completely. The main goals are to reduce the frequency and severity of headaches, lessen their interference with daily life, and improve overall functioning. Progress may be gradual rather than immediate, and treatment may require adjustments over time to determine what works best.

Why? Setting realistic expectations helps patients understand that progress often results in better control. Research shows that patients who view treatment as a process focused on reducing disability, improving quality of life, and gaining coping skills, are more likely to stay engaged, avoid frustration, and adhere to the treatment plan [12].

Case Vignette—Continued

Dr. L: *Thank you for bringing in your headache diary.* [Dr. L reviews the diary]. *Was there anything that you noticed when completing this? A pattern, maybe?* [shares diary with the patient to review together].

Ms. A: *Well.* [pauses] *It looks like I get headaches when I do not sleep well. It happened here, here, and here.* [points to the diary].

Dr. L: *I agree with you! When I look at your log, it appears that the headaches occur after you haven't slept well; thus, you may not sleep well when your head hurts, but poor sleep also seems to be a trigger.*

Ms. A: *You are right. What can we do about my sleep though? Is there a pill or something?*

Dr. L: *Many people notice more headaches with poor sleep. The good news is that sleep can be improved without medications. Before we jump into sleep improvement recommendations, can we look at the rest of the diary to make sure we don't miss any other triggers?*

Ms. A: *Sure! Let's do that.*

Dr. L: *It looks like alcohol may also be a trigger for your headaches. I also see that you tend to have headaches when you are feeling more stressed out. How do you usually cope with your stress?*

Ms. A: *Well, sometimes I have a glass of wine to help me relax!* [laughs]. *Otherwise, I am not sure.*

Dr. L: *Before we go on, do you see what I am seeing?* [points to the diary]. *It looks like every day after you drink wine the headache starts in the morning.*

Ms. A: *I see what you are saying. What do you recommend? I know I am stressed but therapy is not an option for me right now. I have too many things going on. Can we figure out something for the headaches?*

Dr. L: *I know your goal is to have more headache-free days. It looks like we identified three triggers for your headaches—poor sleep, drinking wine, and stress. From a medical point of view, the best way to manage headaches is to avoid triggers altogether, but addressing all three can be tough.*

Ms. A: *It is tough. Can we focus on one?*

Dr. L: *Absolutely! Which one do you want to begin?*

Ms. A: *Maybe stress management? I know wine is not the only answer. What do you recommend?*

Dr. L: *There are multiple ways to reduce stress. I find that many patients benefit from daily mindfulness practice. I can show you a quick mindfulness exercise right now, if you would like.*

Ms. A: *Yes, that would be helpful. I am not really sure how to get started.*

Dr. L: Guides patient through a meditation (see Resources) and provides her with materials for free meditation practice at home. For sleep interventions, see Chap. 5, *Insomnia*. For brief interventions targeting alcohol reduction, refer to Rodgers [31].

Non-pharmacological Treatment Options: What Can Be Done?

Strategies such as identifying headache triggers, managing stress, and promoting physical activity are effective components of headache management and can be easily introduced during a routine **PC** visit [10].

Encourage Patients to Keep a Headache Diary

A headache diary allows patients to record key characteristics (e.g., intensity, location, duration) and supports:

- Identifying patterns and triggers
- Evaluating the impact of lifestyle changes
- Reducing unnecessary medication use
- Improving communication with providers

Why? Headaches are often episodic and subjective, making it difficult to assess patterns without documentation. Consistent **tracking** provides valuable information about treatment effectiveness, particularly for patients with chronic or complex presentations [3]. For tools to support **tracking**, see Resources.

Introduce Relaxation Training as a Behavioral Strategy

Patients may attempt to manage headaches by withdrawing from activities — an approach that can worsen symptoms over time. Instead, physicians can encourage sustainable behavioral strategies that support long-term symptom control. Stress should be normalized as a common trigger, and relaxation practices should be framed as management tools.

Examples of brief relaxation techniques that can be introduced in clinic:

1. Diaphragmatic Breathing: A simple relaxation technique that can help calm the body and reduce headache intensity or frequency:
   (a) Ask the patient to sit comfortably with one hand on their chest and the other just below the rib cage.
   (b) Ask the patient to inhale slowly through the nose for a count of four, allowing the stomach to rise, and then pause.
   (c) Exhale gently through the mouth for a count of six.
   (d) Repeat this pattern for 5 to10 minutes, once or twice a day, or whenever a headache begins.
2. Progressive Muscle Relaxation (PMR)—Short Version: Focuses on reducing tension in areas prone to tightness such as the shoulders and jaw:
   (a) Ask the patient to sit comfortably with hands rested in their lap or at their sides.
   (b) Gently tense each muscle (e.g., shoulders) for a few seconds, then release, noticing the difference between a tense and relaxed muscle.
   (c) Patients can progressively tense and relax other muscle groups throughout the body.

Recommending daily practice of either or both techniques can assist patients with building necessary skills to address the somatic aspects of stress management. See Resources for handouts and apps to support these practices.

Why? Relaxation training, particularly diaphragmatic breathing and PMR, reduces headache frequency and severity while improving patient engagement [34]. Through consistent practice, patients learn to intentionally regulate physiological functions such as muscle tension, heart rate, and breathing [13, 38].

Psychotherapy Effectiveness

Cognitive-behavioral therapy (CBT) is the most well-supported psychotherapeutic intervention for PH [2, 21]. CBT helps patients address relationships among stress, coping, and headache symptoms [28]. While cognitive strategies modify response patterns to symptoms, behavioral strategies support habit modification to improve trigger management.

Meta-analytic reviews consistently demonstrate that behavioral interventions, including **relaxation training**, **biofeedback**, CBT, and stress management, yield a 35 to 55% reduction in **migraine** and **TTH** symptoms, significantly outperforming control conditions [29]. More recent evidence reinforces these findings. In a meta-analysis of 27 randomized controlled trials (RCTs), Lee et al. [21] reported that CBT produced the greatest improvements relative to other psychological interventions (i.e., **biofeedback, relaxation training**, mindfulness-based interventions). When analyzed by type of intervention, CBT was associated with the largest reduction in headache frequency, with a pooled mean difference of −3.00 days (95% CI [−5.43, −0.57]) compared with control groups. By contrast, **biofeedback** showed a smaller effect (−0.70 days, 95% CI [−1.37, −0.02]), and mindfulness-based therapy demonstrated a modest and nonsignificant effect (−1.29 days, 95% CI [−2.13, 0.64]).

Integrative Medicine Interventions and Techniques

Integrative medicine (IM) interventions encompass a range of non-pharmacological treatments that complement standard medical care for headache management. Interventions, such as **biofeedback**, **acupuncture**, **manual therapy,** and **dietary supplements** can reduce headache frequency and severity while improving quality of life.

1. **Biofeedback** helps patients gain voluntary control over physiological processes, such as muscle tension and skin temperature, both of which are often associated with headache onset and intensity. Evidence indicates that **biofeedback** is moderately effective for **TTH** and **migraine,** producing small to moderate reductions in headache frequency ($g = -0.20$, 95% CI: [−0.39, −0.01]), and severity ($g = -0.68$, 95% CI: [−1.07, −0.30]) [27].
2. In a RCT trial examining **acupuncture** for **TTH**, more than half of participants in the treatment group experienced at least 50% reduction in headache frequency. This reduction was both clinically meaningful and statistically significant [23].
3. A review of RCTs indicates that physiotherapy can improve headache frequency, intensity, disability, and quality of life in adults with **TTH**. Physiotherapy approaches, including **manual therapy** techniques such as massage and stretching, demonstrated benefits both post-treatment and at six-month follow-up, with effect sizes of up to 0.62 [6].

4. **Dietary supplements**, specifically magnesium and riboflavin, may help prevent **migraines**. A systematic review and meta-analysis found that magnesium (121.5–600 mg/day) reduced **migraine** attacks by 2.5 per month (mean difference [*MD*] = −2.51), slightly reduced headache severity (*MD* = −0.88), and decreased the number of monthly **migraine** days by 1.7 compared to controls (*MD* = −1.66). Riboflavin at 400 mg/day also significantly reduced **migraine** frequency by 1.3 attacks per month compared with those not taking the supplement (*MD* = −1.34) [37].

Clinical Pearls

- Collaborate with patients to identify biological, behavioral, and psychosocial triggers and develop a personalized, multimodal plan.
- Encourage patients to keep a headache diary that tracks frequency, duration, severity, triggers, medication use, and lifestyle factors (e.g., sleep, exercise, stress) to identify modifiable contributors.
- Incorporate brief relaxation techniques, such as diaphragmatic breathing or PMR exercises, to manage stress—a common headache trigger.
- Consider integrative approaches, including **biofeedback**, mindfulness, **acupuncture**, yoga, massage, or supplements like magnesium or riboflavin, as adjuncts to standard care.
- Set realistic expectations by clarifying that treatment is a process focused on improving quality of life and coping skills rather than achieving a complete cure.

Frequently Asked Questions

Question 1: *Could something I eator drink trigger my headaches?*
Answer: Yes, certain foods and beverages can trigger headaches, particularly **migraines**. Common culprits include alcohol (e.g., red wine), caffeine, aged cheeses, chocolate, and foods containing additives such as monosodium glutamate (MSG). Keeping a headache diary that records intake and headache timing can help identify patterns and potential triggers. Once identified, targeted dietary adjustments may help reduce headache frequency and severity.

Question 2: *Can stress trigger or worsen my headaches?*
Answer: Yes. Stress is one of the most common triggers for **migraines** and **TTH**. Large-scale research shows that over 90% of patients with headaches identify stress as a trigger [9]. Stress can increase muscle tension, alter blood flow, and heighten pain sensitivity, contributing to headache onset or worsening. Managing stress through techniques such as relaxation exercises, mindfulness, or structured therapies like MBSR has been shown to reduce headache frequency and severity.

Question 3: *I've cut caffeine, sleep more, exercise, and still get headaches. What do I do now?*

Answer: If headaches persist, your **PC** doctor may review the diagnosis, rule out other causes (e.g., sleep apnea or jaw/neck issues), and consider referral to a specialist. Treatment often combines lifestyle changes, medication, and stress management therapies. While these approaches may not eliminate headaches, they can reduce severity and improve overall control. The goal is improved management, rather than an immediate cure.

Resources

Source	Description	Link
Patient education resources		
National Headache Foundation	Educational information, headache diary, diet guide, podcast, and videos	https://headaches.org
National Headache Foundation	Educational information on causes, types, triggers, and management of headaches in Spanish	https://headaches.org/category/headache-fact-sheets-spanish/?utm_source=chatgpt.com
National Headache Foundation—Low Tyramine Headache Diet	Brief printable PDF guide to low tyramine dietary options	https://headaches.org/wp-content/uploads/2025/05/Low-Tyramine-Diet-0525.pdf
Headache tracking tools		
N1-Headache	Free app that offers tracking of symptoms and triggers	https://n1-headache.com/
Migraine Buddy	Free app that offers tracking of symptoms and triggers	https://migrainebuddy.com/what-is-migraine-buddy-free-and-easy-migraine-tracker/
Usar Migraine Buddy	Free app that offers tracking of symptoms and triggers in Spanish	https://migrainebuddy.com/es/categor%C3%ADa/usar-migraine-buddy/
National Headache Foundation	Printable headache diary	https://headaches.org/wp-content/uploads/2021/05/HEADACHE-DIARY.pdf
Kaiser Permanente	Printable headache diary in Spanish	https://mydoctor.kaiserpermanente.org/ncal/Images/HeadacheDiarySPAN_tcm75-1439796.pdf
Therapy and mindfulness resources		
Click Therapeutics	A prescription digital therapeutic app offering evidence-based behavioral techniques	https://www.clicktherapeutics.com/products/ct-132
Centre for Clinical Intervention	Printable PMR exercise	Information-SheetsProgressive-Muscle-Relaxation.pdf
Headspace	Free app that offers guided meditations and educational animations	https://www.headspace.com/

(continued)

Source	Description	Link
Smiling Mind	Free app that offers guided meditations and age-specific content	https://www.smilingmind.com.au/
Bilingual Center for Mindfulness	Offers free guided meditations and mindfulness exercises in Spanish	https://bilingualmindfulness.com/

Case Vignette—Conclusion

Ms. A returns for her one-month follow-up with her headache diary.

Ms. A: *I still have some headaches but get them less often. I wish I still didn't get these many headaches though.*

Dr. L: [Reviews headache diary.] *I see that you are having fewer headaches more recently compared to when you first started* ***tracking*** *your headaches and symptoms.* [Points to diary] *Do you notice any patterns?*

Ms. A: *I have fewer days when I marked that I was stressed, and fewer days with headaches.*

Dr. L: *I see that! What do you make of that?*

Ms. A: *I have been practicing meditation most evenings using the free app you showed me, and I have felt a little less stressed.*

Dr. L: *How do you feel you are progressing toward your goal of having more headache-free days?*

Ms. A: *I am having more days without headaches now, but I still feel I have too many. Is there something natural I can take to stop having so many headaches?*

Dr. L: *A supplement that may help reduce the frequency of your headaches and has minimal side effects is riboflavin. You can start taking riboflavin 400 mg/day in addition to continuing to practice meditation. Please continue* ***tracking*** *your symptoms with the headache diary so we can check in in about one month. How does that sound?*

Ms. A: *That sounds good.*

References

1. Alaqeel AM, Alaqeel SS, Andijani AI, Demyati EA. Validity and reliability of an Arabic version of the migraine screen questionnaire in the primary care setting for identifying hidden migraine. Int J Med Developing Countries. 2021;5(3):906–10. https://doi.org/10.24911/IJMDC.51.1611922218.
2. Amatrudo G, Kengetter J, McCrea S, Amatrudo M. Cognitive behavioral therapy for the management of episodic migraine. Curr Pain Headache Rep. 2023;27(9):471–7. https://doi.org/10.1007/s11916-023-01129-y.
3. American Migraine Foundation. Keeping a headache diary. 2022. https://americanmigrainefoundation.org/resource-library/keeping-a-headache-diary/.
4. Balasubramanian B, Nair VS, George N, Reddy AV, Thomas PT, Kulkarni GB. A bio-psychosocial framework for chronic daily headaches: a mixed methods study. J Patient Exp. 2021;8:23743735211049672. https://doi.org/10.1177/23743735211049672.

5. Burch R, Rizzoli P, Loder E. The prevalence and impact of migraine and severe headache in the United States: figures and trends from government health studies. Headache. 2018;58(4):496–505. https://doi.org/10.1111/head.13281.
6. Chaibi A, Russell MB. Manual therapies for primary chronic headaches: a systematic review of randomized controlled trials. J Headache Pain. 2014;15(1):67. https://doi.org/10.1186/1129-2377-15-67.
7. Do TP, Remmers A, Schytz HW, Schankin C, Nelson SE, Obermann M, Hansen JM, Sinclair AJ, Gantenbein AR, Schoonman GG. Red and orange flags for secondary headaches in clinical practice: SNNOOP10 list. Neurology. 2019;92(3):134–44. https://doi.org/10.1212/WNL.0000000000006697.
8. Elbadawi ASA, Albalawi AFA, Alghannami AK, Alsuhaymi FS, Alruwaili AM, Almaleki FA, Almutairi MF, Almubaddil KH, Qashqari MI. Cluster headache and associated risk factors: a systematic review and meta-analysis. Cureus. 2021;13(11):e19294. https://doi.org/10.7759/cureus.19294.
9. Elmazny A, Magdy R, Hussein M, Ismaeel AY, Essmat A, Elbeltagy KE, Hussein SMM, Hassan NS, Elbehiry NM, Osama W, Abdelazeem HN, Elshebawy H. Migraine triggers and lifestyle modifications: an assessment of patients' awareness and the role of healthcare providers in patient education. J Headache Pain. 2025;26(1):189. https://doi.org/10.1186/s10194-025-02107-y.
10. Ford B, Dore M, Harris E. Outpatient primary care management of headaches: guidelines from the VA/DoD. Am Fam Physician. 2021;104(3):316–20.
11. Gagnon KW, Quinn K, Walsh JL, Amirkhanian YA, Kelly JA. Characteristics of healthcare providers, healthcare systems, and patient strategies related to medical mistrust among black and African Americans. BMC Prim Care. 2025;26(1):203. https://doi.org/10.1186/s12875-025-02900-3.
12. Gaul C, Liesering-Latta E, Schäfer B, Fritsche G, Holle D. Integrated multidisciplinary care of headache disorders: a narrative review. Cephalalgia. 2016;36(12):1181–91. https://doi.org/10.1177/0333102415617413.
13. Gopichandran L, Srivastsava AK, Vanamail P, Kanniammal C, Valli G, Mahendra J, Dhandapani M. Effectiveness of progressive muscle relaxation and deep breathing exercise on pain, disability, and sleep among patients with chronic tension-type headache: a randomized control trial. Holist Nurs Pract. 2024;38(5):285–96. https://doi.org/10.1097/hnp.0000000000000460.
14. Hussein M, Hassan A, Nada MAF, Mohammed Z, Abdel Ghaffar NF, Kedah H, Fathy W, Magdy R. Reliability, validity, and responsiveness of the Arabic version of HIT-6 questionnaire in patients with migraine indicated for preventive therapy: a multi-center study. Headache. 2024;64(5):500–8. https://doi.org/10.1111/head.14719.
15. Headache Classification Committee of the International Headache Society (IHS) The International Classification of Headache Disorders, 3rd edition. Cephalalgia: An International Journal of Headache. 2018;38(1):1–211.
16. Kandel SA, Mandiga P. Cluster headache. In: StatPearls. StatPearls Publishing; 2023. https://www.ncbi.nlm.nih.gov/books/NBK544241/.
17. Kennis K, Kernick D, O'Flynn N. Diagnosis and management of headaches in young people and adults: NICE guideline. Br J Gen Pract. 2013;63(613):443–5. https://doi.org/10.3399/bjgp13X670895.
18. Kiarashi J, VanderPluym J, Szperka CL, Turner S, Minen MT, Broner S, Ross AC, Wagstaff AE, Anto M, Marzouk M, Monteith TS, Rosen N, Manrriquez SL, Seng E, Finkel A, Charleston L IV. Factors associated with, and mitigation strategies for health care disparities faced by patients with headache disorders. Neurology. 2021;97(6):280–9. https://doi.org/10.1212/WNL.0000000000012261.
19. Kikkeri NS, Nagalli S. Trigeminal neuralgia. In: StatPearls. StatPearls Publishing; 2024. https://www.ncbi.nlm.nih.gov/books/NBK554486.

20. Lang AC, Igler EC, Linneman NG, Brimeyer CT, Drendel AL, Davies WH. Practice recommendations for contextualizing explanations of headache pain within a biopsychosocial model. Patient Educ Couns. 2025;137:109175. https://doi.org/10.1016/j.pec.2025.109175.
21. Lee HJ, Lee JH, Cho EY, Kim SM, Yoon S. Efficacy of psychological treatment for headache disorder: a systematic review and meta-analysis. J Headache Pain. 2019;20(1):17. https://doi.org/10.1186/s10194-019-0965-4.
22. Ličina E, Radojicic A, Jeremic M, Tomic A, Mijajlovic M. Non-pharmacological treatment of primary headaches—a focused review. Brain Sci. 2023;13(10):1432. https://doi.org/10.3390/brainsci13101432.
23. Linde K, Allais G, Brinkhaus B, Fei Y, Mehring M, Shin BC, Vickers A, White AR. Acupuncture for the prevention of tension-type headache. Cochrane Database Syst Rev. 2016;4(4):CD007587. https://doi.org/10.1002/14651858.CD007587.pub2.
24. Lipton RB, Dodick D, Sadovsky R, Kolodner K, Endicott J, Hettiarachchi J, Harrison W. A self-administered screener for migraine in primary care: the ID Migraine™ validation study. Neurology. 2003;61(3):375–82. https://doi.org/10.1212/01.WNL.0000078940.53438.83.
25. Mapi Research Trust Migraine Disability Assessment (MIDAS). 2025. https://eprovide.mapi-trust.org/instruments/migraine-disability-assessment#basic_description.
26. Mourad D, Hajj A, Hallit S, Ghossoub M, Khabbaz LR. Validation of the Arabic version of the Migraine Disability Assessment Scale among Lebanese patients with migraine. J Oral Facial Pain Headache. 2019;33(1):47–53. https://doi.org/10.11607/ofph.2102.
27. Paudel P, Sah A. Efficacy of biofeedback for migraine: a systematic review and meta-analysis. Complement Ther Med. 2025;58:102736. https://doi.org/10.1016/j.ctim.2025.102736.
28. Penzien DB, Irby MB, Smitherman TA, Rains JC, Houle TT. Well-established and empirically supported behavioral treatments for migraine. Curr Pain Headache Rep. 2015;19(7):34. https://doi.org/10.1007/s11916-015-0500-5.
29. Rains JC, Penzien DB, McCrory DC, Gray RN. Behavioral headache treatment: history, review of the empirical literature, and methodological critique. Headache. 2005;45(Suppl. 2):S92–S109. https://doi.org/10.1111/j.1526-4610.2005.4502003.x.
30. Rendas-Baum R, Yang M, Varon SF, Bloudek LM, DeGryse RE, Kosinski M. Validation of the Headache Impact Test (HIT-6) in patients with chronic migraine. Health Qual Life Outcomes. 2014;12:117. https://doi.org/10.1186/s12955-014-0117-0.
31. Rodgers C. Brief interventions for alcohol and other drug use. Aust Prescr. 2018;41(4):117–21. https://doi.org/10.18773/austprescr.2018.031.
32. Rodríguez-Almagro D, Achalandabaso A, Rus A, Obrero-Gaitán E, Zagalaz-Anula N, Lomas-Vega R. Validation of the Spanish version of the migraine disability assessment questionnaire (MIDAS) in university students with migraine. BMC Neurol. 2020;20(1):67. https://doi.org/10.1186/s12883-020-01646-y.
33. Rodríguez-Rivas R, Moreno-Martínez CA, Cerqueira TL, Enríquez-Peregrino KG, Martínez-Piña DA, Vargas-Rodríguez JN, Zermeño F. Translation, cross-cultural adaptation, and validation of the ID Migraine™ screening test into Latin American Spanish. Headache. 2023;63(7):843–5. https://doi.org/10.1111/head.14509.
34. Seng EK, Holroyd KA. Behavioral migraine management modifies behavioral and cognitive coping in people with migraine. Headache. 2014;54(9):1470–83. https://doi.org/10.1111/head.12426.
35. Stewart WF, Lipton RB, Whyte J, Dowson A, Kolodner K, Liberman JN, Sawyer J. An international study to assess reliability of the Migraine Disability Assessment (MIDAS) score. Neurology. 1999;53(5):988–94. https://doi.org/10.1212/wnl.53.5.988.
36. Stewart WF, Lipton RB, Dowson AJ. Development and testing of the Migraine Disability Assessment (MIDAS) Questionnaire. Neurology. 2001;56(6 Suppl 1):S20–8. https://doi.org/10.1212/wnl.56.suppl_1.s20.
37. Talandashti MK, Shahinfar H, Delgarm P, Jazayeri S. Effects of selected dietary supplements on migraine prophylaxis: a systematic review and dose-response meta-analysis of randomized controlled trials. Neurol Sci. 2025;46(2):651–70. https://doi.org/10.1007/s10072-024-07794-0.

38. Toussaint L, Nguyen QA, Roettger C, Dixon K, Offenbächer M, Kohls N, Hirsch J, Sirois F. Effectiveness of progressive muscle relaxation, deep breathing, and guided imagery in promoting psychological and physiological states of relaxation. Evid Based Complement Alternat Med. 2021;2021:5924040. https://doi.org/10.1155/2021/5924040.
39. Viera AJ, Antono B. Acute headache in adults: a diagnostic approach. Am Fam Physician. 2022;106(3):260–8. https://www.aafp.org/pubs/afp/issues/2022/0900/acute-headache-adults.html.
40. Wang X, Sun J, Xing Y, Zhou H, Zhao Y. Validation of the Chinese version of the Identification of Migraine Screener (ID Migraine) in university students in Harbin, China. J Oral Facial Pain Headache. 2015;29(4):384–6. https://doi.org/10.11607/ofph.1341.

Chapter 10
Understanding Psychotherapy Services: Crash Course for Physicians

Nataliya Pilipenko

Introduction

It is estimated that 23% of adults in the US live with a mental illness [36]. In primary care (PC), one in nine encounters (11.7%) involves a mental-health complaint [11].

Communication Training Gaps

While communication skills are recognized as a central training and practice competency for physicians in the U.S., currently medical education "lacks overarching standards and certification" [37, p. 151]. Additionally, although biopsychosocial formulation and inquiry is central to addressing both physical and psychiatric chronic health concerns, it is often overlooked in PC [33]. Moreover, physicians receive limited training and report low comfort when counseling patients presenting with psychiatric conditions [20, 22]. For example, Alhawshani and colleagues [1] report that while 86% residents completed a mental health-related rotation, just 61% received didactic training and only 28% received **psychotherapy supervision**. Overall training was limited to 5 hours or less. By contrast, licensed psychologists in the US are required to complete at least 5 years of academic training (which includes extensive study of psychopathology, psychotherapeutics, and clinical

N. Pilipenko (✉)
Center for Family and Community Medicine, Department of Medicine, Columbia University Irving Medical Center/New York Presbyterian Hospital, New York, NY, USA

Department of Psychiatry, Columbia University Irving Medical Center, New York, NY, USA
e-mail: np2615@cumc.columbia.edu

N. Pilipenko, K. M. Desai (eds.), *8 Conditions Primary Care Clinicians Dread to Treat*, https://doi.org/10.1007/978-3-032-12819-5_10

skills) as well as 3500 hours of supervision during doctoral training and 1750 hours of supervision after completion of doctoral studies [45].

While research indicates that "efforts should be made to better identify, clarify, and improve physicians' counseling skills" [20] it is not clear whether, when, and how this can be achieved. Thus, improved understanding of factors implicated in effective referrals, partnership, and support of **psychotherapy engagement** appear important for addressing psychiatric treatment needs within PC. In order for this to be accomplished, PC physicians must possess understanding of factors implicated in both effective and ineffective **psychotherapy** care.

This chapter aims to improve physicians' understanding of factors that are central to the delivery of **evidence-based psychotherapy (EBP)** care. However, it does not address specialty testing (e.g., personality, developmental, forensic, disability, neuropsychological, etc.) since these are governed by a unique set of rules and regulations and require in depth discussion. For guidance on these areas, see Institute of Medicine's overview of psychological testing for disability determination [13], American Psychological Association's specialty guidelines for forensic psychology [2], American Academy of Clinical Neuropsychology's practice guidelines for neuropsychological assessment and consultation [10] and other relevant sources.

Why Should Physicians Care About Their Patients' Psychotherapy Treatment?

Connections between psychiatric and medical conditions are complex. However, there are two key reasons why physicians (even those who do not directly treat psychiatric illness) can benefit from understanding psychiatric concerns.

Comorbid Psychiatric Conditions Negatively Impact Physical Health

Epidemiologic data that suggests patients with psychiatric illnesses are expected to die 15–20 years earlier than those without such conditions, with 70% of these deaths attributable to medical causes [6].

Momen et al. [34] note that "most mental disorders were associated with an increased risk of a subsequent medical condition" and there is a growing body of research supporting psychiatric pathology as a risk factor for physical health. For example, depression, posttraumatic stress disorder (PTSD), and anxiety disorders are linked to the development and progression of cardiovascular disease [12]. Panic attacks predict emergence of asthma [23], while chronic sleep problems are associated with increased rates of hypertension, diabetes, obesity, depression, heart attack, and stroke [27]. Thus, failure to adequately address psychiatric illness is likely to negatively impact medical outcomes.

Psychotherapy Interventions Improve Physical Illness Outcomes

There is a growing body of literature which supports effectiveness of **EBP** interventions for improved outcome for physical illnesses (with or without psychiatric comorbidities). For example, protocols are available for:

1. Various pain conditions such as chronic pain, headache, rheumatologic pain, chronic back pain, fibromyalgia, irritable bowel syndrome (see American Psychological Association, Society of Clinical Psychology resource for detailed information)
2. Hypertension [29]
3. Diabetes mellitus [30]
4. Asthma [28]
5. Cardiac health issues [26]

Many approaches are culturally adapted and/or include components which address psychiatric comorbidities. For example, Feldman and colleagues [18] report significant improvements in reduction of panic symptom severity, improved asthma control, and increased medication adherence among a sample of Latino adults following only eight sessions of culturally adapted **cognitive behavioral therapy**. Therefore, it is important for physicians to be aware of the value which **EBP** can bring to treatment of different medical conditions seen within PC.

What Is Evidence-Based Psychotherapy Practice?

According to the American Psychological Association [5], **psychotherapy** is a service provided by a trained professional to an individual or group of individuals (e.g., couples, families) whereby "communication and interaction [are used to] assess, diagnose, and treat dysfunctional emotional reactions, ways of thinking, and behavior patterns."

Evidence-based practice (**EBP**) of **psychotherapy** follows the same principles as the evidence-based practice of medicine. Specifically, **EBP** involves "conscientious, explicit, and judicious use of current best evidence in making decisions about care of individual patients" [42]. Thus, **EBP** implementation aims for "mindful integration of both scientific evidence (e.g., research studies) and local evidence (e.g., situational assessments) often with the help of decision supports" [41].

Overarchingly, **EBPs** share four key features:

1. *Demonstrated effectiveness.* There is substantial body of evidence indicating that a specific approach significantly reduces symptoms and/or improves patients' quality of life.
2. *Goal directedness.* Goals of treatment are set at the start of the treatment and are used to guide both interventions and evaluation of the progress.
3. *Time limits.* **EBP** are typically delivered within 12–20 sessions, although some approaches, such as behavioral activation can be delivered in as few as four sessions.
4. *Lasting benefits.* Treatment gains should be maintained over time. This is predicated on **psychotherapy** being an active process whereby a patient learns and applies skills to address identified problems.

It is important that PC physicians are cognizant of **EBP** features when considering referrals and evaluating whether the patient is benefiting from care.

EBP Limitations

Cook and colleagues [14] summarize the following limitations to **EBPs**:

1. *Generalizability.* Validity of **EBP**s outside of the research settings and for groups which were not included in the research studying EBPs' effectiveness may be limited.
2. *Alignment of goals.* While **EBP**s focus on symptom reductions, patients seeking therapy may not conceptualize their difficulties in the same manner.
3. *Alignment with existing practice/training.* **EBP**s are primarily **CBT**- based while many practicing psychotherapists received limited **CBT** training or prioritize other approaches (e.g., psychodynamic).
4. *Appropriate **EBP** may not be available.* There may be a lack of **EBP** for a specific concern or there is insufficient evidence to support **psychotherapy** interventions.
5. *Overlooking clinical experience.* Overly rigid adherence to **EBP**s may raise concerns about insufficient regard for therapists' clinical judgement and flexibility of interventions.
6. *Training burden.* Certification and continuing education may pose a significant burden on therapists.

It is important to note that despite **EBP**'s limitations, current professional organizations and regulatory bodies emphasize the role of **EBP** in the delivery of highest level of clinical practice.

Cognitive Behavioral Therapy: Current "Gold Standard" of EBP

Cognitive behavioral therapy (CBT) is the current "gold standard" for **EBP**—it underwent the most research scrutiny, consistently demonstrated superiority compared to other psychotherapies while its mechanisms and principles are both extensively studied and align with current paradigms of behavior and cognition [15]. Gaudiano [21] notes it is most appropriate to refer to cognitive behavioral therapies in the plural, as **CBT**s constitute a family of related interventions that are grounded in shared principles and assumptions.

Specifically, there are three interconnected "waves" of **CBT**: the first wave (behavioral therapy) is grounded in principles of classical and operant conditioning; the second wave (cognitive therapy), focuses on addressing thinking patterns and beliefs, exemplified by work of Aaron Beck [7], and Albert Ellis [16]; lastly, the third wave which includes Acceptance and Commitment Therapy [25], Dialectical Behavioral Therapy [31] and Mindfulness Based **CBT** [43]. Third wave **CBT**s build on the first and second waves but focus on "mindfulness, emotions, acceptance, the therapeutic relationship, values, goals, and meta-cognition" [24]. These "waves" are complementary and build on each other, and no single "wave" is necesserily superior to others.

Example of a Typical CBT Session

A typical session begins with a symptom check to assess patient's functioning. An agenda is then set, followed by updates and review of the between-sessions tasks (i.e., homework). The therapist then introduces information about new concepts (psychoeducation), subsequently patient and therapist engage in a collaborative discussion about the topic, new between-session tasks are agreed upon, and any potential barriers are discussed. Before the end of the visit, the therapist elicits patient's feedback about the session to support collaboration and active treatment engagement (adapted from [8]).

Basic Processes of EBPs: What Can Be Expected?

Although various EBPs are currently available. There are several commonalities shared by all approaches. These include:

Step 1. Assessment and Differential Diagnostics: To deliver a treatment, a patient's symptoms, antecedents, and maintaining factors need to be assessed and communicated to them. Diagnostic impressions are discussed with the patient to ensure clarity, understanding, and agreement.

Step 2. Treatment selection and planning: For many conditions, multiple **EBPs** may be available. For example, both behavioral activation and cognitive therapy have strong research support for depression treatment [44]. Additionally, given the prevalence of psychiatric comorbidities, the patient is likely to experience several conditions, in which case, priority of treatment efforts should be established. Overall, treatment selection incorporates: best fit and patient's preferences, therapist's training, and settings. Question of settings may be particularly salient, as certain conditions including severe eating disorders, substance use disorders, severe mental illness such as schizophrenia as well as certain personality disorders (e.g., borderline personality disorder) may not be appropriate for treatment by a therapist practicing outside of a specialty team/service. Upon starting **EBP**, goals, duration, and expectations should be discussed with the patient to facilitate engagement as part of the informed consent.

Step 3. Delivery of EBP include the following:

A. Ongoing patient education about diagnosis, factors and mechanisms which maintain it, and processes by which a patient should expect to achieve symptom reduction.
B. Skills building during the visit: these may be behavioral such as diaphragmatic breathing, cognitive such as learning to examine own perceptions (e.g., cognitive disputation), emotional, and/or interpersonal.
C. Skills application outside of the visit: plans are typically set to guide the patient's independent, in vivo application of the skills discussed in session.
D. Problem solving: patients are bound to experience challenges and setbacks during the course of treatment. Addressing ongoing and emerging problems is intrinsic to the **psychotherapy** process.
E. Assessment of progress towards goal: Since **EBP**s are goal directed, regular review of progress is essential. It is important to note that patients should not remain in **psychotherapy treatment** when they are not benefitting or are being harmed [4].

Step 4. Termination

The final stage of treatment includes focusing on the consolidation of treatment gains, relapse prevention planning, and overview of the progress made. Termination is an important treatment process. While termination can be dictated by external factors (e.g., insurance coverage), patients should be clear about anticipated duration of treatment and follow up plan (e.g., availability of booster sessions, referrals to alternative sources).

Ineffective and Problematic Psychotherapy: "Red Flags"

Patients treated by PC physicians may present for care expressing frustration with lack of symptom relief in their **psychotherapy treatment**. It is important to remember that **psychotherapy** progress requires time, and some level of difficulty is to be expected even in successful **EBP** implementation. However, several "**red flags**" can alert physicians to problems within the **psychotherapy** process. These include:

1. Patient is unaware of the diagnosis or is unable to describe treatment method/process of change.

Why is this a problem? Delivery of **EBP** is based on the patient's understanding of the problem which is encapsulated by the diagnosis. Diagnostic conceptualization informs patients of the unique "footprint" of the diagnosis and informs treatment planning and goal setting. **EBPs** have unique components for each disorder of focus. For example, patients with posttraumatic stress disorder receive different interventions than those suffering from panic disorder. If the patient is unable to understand diagnosis and treatment process, this raises concerns about their ability to participate in care. To better evaluate these aspects, consider asking:

(a) What is the diagnosis for which you are getting **psychotherapy**?
(b) Did your therapist talk to you about their approach? (If so) What is your understanding of the process? What steps will you take to improve your [symptoms]?
(c) What are some of the treatment goals for your **psychotherapy**? What skills are you learning to help you achieve these?

2. The patient describes **psychotherapy** sessions as "We just speak about things that are going on."

Why is this a problem? EBPs protocols have a tight focus with each session aiming to deliver new information and support new skills acquisition. While not every session can be delivered in adherence with stringent guidelines, overall, this structure aims to reduce patient's suffering in least time possible and allow for the clinical resource (i.e., psychotherapist's time which is typically supported via insurance billing) to be available to the maximum number of patients. Treatment without goals, aims, purpose, and strategies needs to be critically appraised from an ethical perspective.

Physician may ask the following questions to clarify treatment goals:

(a) Do you believe that your therapy is helping you to reduce symptoms of [psychiatric condition]?
(b) Are there techniques or strategies that you learned in therapy which help you to deal with 'things that are going on'?
(c) Do you and your therapist discuss how long you will be in treatment for? How you will address [symptoms] once your treatment is completed?

3. Patient expects their individual **psychotherapy** to change others' behaviors.

Why is this a problem? The process of **psychotherapy** is unable to target behaviors of persons who are not involved in it. While patients can reasonably expect to learn improved ways of relating with others (i.e., via assertive communication or anger management techniques), the focus of treatment needs to remain on the patient. Patients seeking treatment with the primary goal of changing behaviors of others (e.g., adult children, spouses) should be advised to consider couples or family, rather than individual **psychotherapy**.

4. Patient Reports relationships with their therapist outside of the therapeutic relationship (e.g., romantic/sexual, socializing, gift giving)

Why is this a problem? Psychotherapy delivery is governed by a specific set of ethical rules which aim to protect the patient from being exploited or mistreated. For example, practicing psychologists in the US, are prohibited from engaging in sexual relationships with current patients or current patients' relatives or significant others, are not allowed to provide therapy to former sexual partners, and are prohibited from engaging in sexual relations with former patients for at least 2 years [3].

As patients are in a vulnerable state during treatment, they may have difficulties in recognizing and addressing therapist's inappropriate behavior. Moreover, patients might themselves initiate situations whereby ethical considerations emerge (e.g., give expensive gifts, initiate social contact online). Furthermore, specifics of behaviors which constitute prohibited conduct may differ between professionals who deliver **psychotherapy**, may depend on geography of practice, and may be defined differently across different codes of professional conduct. The following steps aim to support physicians who have concerns about a patient's report related to **psychotherapy engagement**.

(a) Appropriate documentation outlining patient's report of the concerns and behaviors is necessary. This can subsequently be used to protect the patient and the physician if any legal action should ensue.
(b) Seek consultation. This can be done within the department/institution or directly with the State's licensing board. Many unethical practices can fall on a spectrum and/or evolve over time. Moreover, reporting requirements can differ between States. Thus, consulting to clarify one's own scope of responsibility is critical.
(c) (If appropriate and indicated) Discuss concerns with the patient and develop a plan to support.

Supporting Psychotherapy Engagement: What Can Physicians Do?

Effective ability to refer patients for **psychotherapy** is subject to multiple physician, patient, and system-level factors. This section summarizes physician behaviors which can support this process.

Engage in Holistic, Biopsychosocially-Informed Practice of Medicine

Biopsychosocial conceptualization highlights the interconnectedness between social, psychological, and behavioral dimensions of medical illnesses [17]. This holistic approach allows for integration of various interventions (including and not limited to **psychotherapy**) within treatment and is considered fundamental to PC training and practice. However, McDaniel et al. [32] note that the "split biopsychosocial" model is often practiced in PC: biomedical explanations and treatments are used as the first and sole explanations at the start of the treatment and when these interventions fail to deliver results, physicians fall back on biopsychosocial explanations. Understandably, such shifts undermine patient engagement and satisfaction. Thus, to successfully support engagement, physicians need to routinely frame care as a holistic process whereby multiple approaches can be used in concert to treat illness and support health.

Manage Patient Expectations

While **EBP** care is a collaborative process whereby most of the progress is set in motion by the synergy of factors, no approach will be effective unless the patient presents for care and is actively engaged. Explicitly discussing these expectations with the patient can avoid unnecessary **psychotherapy referral**s. When referring patient for **psychotherapy**, following factors should be discussed to set expectations.

Regular and Timely Attendance

It is important that a patient is able and willing to commit to regular attendance of psychotherapy sessions. Typically, weekly participation would be expected, and patients will be disenrolled from **psychotherapy** service if they miss multiple appointments. Moreover, most psychotherapy visits are billed by time (typically 30–60 min) thus if the patient does not present on time, they are unlikely to be seen for the entire duration of the session (or at all). This factor may be important to consider with patients who have difficulties with punctuality. While the PC model of care delivery may be more flexible to delays, typically more stringent boundaries are applied to **psychotherapy** delivery.

Active Participation

Patients will be asked to engage in discussion and practice techniques both within and between psychotherapy sessions. While therapists will assist patients to address barriers to completing practice tasks outside of sessions, most work is in fact done between visits rather than within patient-therapist meetings. Patients who attend EBT with expectations to feel better quickly while simply "chatting" with their therapist during the session are likely to be disappointed.

Referrals and Partnerships

Typically, when a patient is seeking **psychotherapy**, physicians may provide external or internal referrals. However, patients can enroll into therapy without a PC physician's referral, thus referrals may not be necessary. This may be different for many other services (e.g., specialist referrals, physical therapy). If internal referral for **psychotherapy** is unavailable or somehow inappropriate, the following options can be explored:

1. **Consulting Insurance Carrier**. Ask patient to contact their insurance carrier and request contact information for available in network therapists.
2. **Use Reputable Search Engines**. There are multiple national, State, organizational, or practice specific online resources that provide information about available clinics, services, and therapists. Familiarity with such options is valuable to PC physicians, especially if internal supports (e.g., integrated mental health services, social work teams) are limited or unavailable. See Table 10.1 for information.
3. **Review Past Psychotherapy Efforts**. If a patient successfully engaged in therapy in the past, the best option may be to re-engage with a former therapist or service (e.g., hospital, clinic). This will avoid fragmentation of services and limit the burden of referrals. Consider asking, "Are you able to re-engage with your last therapist/practice site? Do you see any barriers for doing so?"

Table 10.1 Evidence based psychotherapy resources

Resource	Link	Description
U.S Department of Veterans Affairs	https://www.mentalhealth.va.gov/get-help/treatment/ebt.asp	General brief overview of common **EBP**s Including: Duration, anticipated changes, patient expectations
American Psychological Association, Society of Clinical Psychology	https://www.apa.org/about/division/div12	Provides information about evidence-supported psychotherapies for a range of medical and psychiatric conditions. Reviews strength of evidence for relevant psychotherapeutic approaches For each therapy/condition provides relevant publications, treatment manuals and patient resources
Psychology Today	https://www.psychologytoday.com/	Includes information by state/Zip code for following: Psychotherapists, psychiatrists, treatment centers, support groups Allows to filter results by various parameters (e.g, in person/remote, specialties, insurance accepted, therapy types etc).
988	https://988lifeline.org	Crisis support line available 24/7/365. Services via call, chat, text, for hearing impaired.
American Board of Professional Psychology ABPP	https://abpp.org	Offers search feature to locate specialist (board certified) psychologists across a range of sub-specialties including but not limited to: addiction, clinical child and adolescent, couples and family, rehabilitation, geropsychology

Participation in Multiple Psychotherapies

Prior to offering **psychotherapy**, physicians should inquire about a patient's current/ongoing **psychotherapy engagement**. Patients should not be referred for a second, concurrent treatment to target the same psychiatric concern. For example, a patient should not be referred for depression treatment at a community-based site if they are already seeing a therapist in private practice. While patients may be unaware of such restrictions, duplication of **psychotherapy** services raises both ethical and billing/insurance coverage concerns. This limitation does not apply, however, if care is sought for distinct concerns. For example, a patient may be referred for **EBP** of PTSD (for example Prolonged Exposure treatment) while concurrently attending a group to maintain sobriety. When unsure, physicians should inform patients about duplication of service concerns and request that patients discuss these concerns with their current and prospective therapists.

Reason for Referral and Ongoing Communication

Given considerations outlined in **EBP** Treatment Selection and Planning section (see Basic Processes of **EBPs**: What Can be Expected?), it is best to limit the **psychotherapy referral** to a brief outline of the presenting concern (e.g., depressed mood, panic attacks) and any relevant factors (e.g., current stressors, past trauma) rather than indicating recommended treatment approach (e.g., **CBT**i for insomnia).

Furthermore, physicians should familiarize themselves with State and institutional requirements for referral/release of information documentation as these may differ depending on multiple factors. Finally, seeking patients' consent to establish a channel of communication with psychotherapists is central to ensuring that coordinated and holistic care delivery.

References

1. Alhawshani S, Furmli S, Shuvra MMR, Malick A, Dunn LB, Ogrodniczuk JS, Monavvari AA. Psychotherapy for patients with mental health concerns in primary care. Can Fam Physician. 2019;65(10):689–90.
2. American Psychological Association. Specialty guidelines for forensic psychology. 2013. https://www.apa.org/pubs/journals/features/forensic-psychology.pdf.
3. American Psychological Association. Ethical principles of psychologists & code of conduct (2002, Amended June 1, 2010 & January 1, 2017). 2017a. https://www.apa.org/ethics/code.
4. American Psychological Association. Clinical practice guideline for the treatment of PTSD. 2017b. https://www.apa.org/ptsd-guideline/treatments.
5. American Psychological Association. Psychotherapy. n.d. https://www.apa.org/topics/psychotherapy.
6. Austin HA. Chronic physical health conditions & mental illness. Medicine. 2024;52(9):557–60. https://www.sciencedirect.com/science/article/abs/pii/S1357303924001749.
7. Beck AT. Thinking & depression: theory & therapy. Arch Gen Psychiatry. 1964;10:561–71.
8. Beck JS. Chapter 5: the evaluation session. In: Cognitive behavior therapy: basics & beyond. 3rd ed. Guilford press; 2021. p. 71–86.
9. Bilet T, Olsen T, Andersen JR, et al. Cognitive behavioral group therapy for panic disorder in a general clinical setting: a prospective cohort study with 12 to 31-years follow-up. BMC Psychiatry. 2020;20:259. https://doi.org/10.1186/s12888-020-02679-w.
10. Board of Directors. American academy of clinical neuropsychology (AACN) practice guidelines for neuropsychological assessment and consultation. Clin neuropsychol. 2007;21(2): 209–31. https://doi.org/10.1080/13825580601025932.
11. Caspi A, Houts RM, Moffitt TE, et al. A nationwide analysis of 350 million patient encounters reveals a high volume of mental-health conditions in primary care. Nat Ment Health. 2024;2:1208–16. https://doi.org/10.1038/s44220-024-00310-5.
12. Cohen BE, Edmondson D, Kronish IM. State of the art review: depression, stress, anxiety, & cardiovascular disease. Am J Hypertens. 2015;28(11):1295–302. https://doi.org/10.1093/ajh/hpv047.
13. Committee on Psychological Testing, Including Validity Testing, for Social Security Administration Disability Determinations, Board on the Health of Select Populations, & Institute of Medicine. Psychological testing in the service of disability determination (Ch. 3, Overview of Psychological Testing). National Academies Press; 2015. https://www.ncbi.nlm.nih.gov/books/NBK305233/.

14. Cook SC, Schwartz AC, Kaslow NJ. Evidence-based psychotherapy: advantages & challenges. Neurotherapeutics. 2017;14(3):537–45. https://doi.org/10.1007/s13311-017-0549-4.
15. David D, Cristea I, Hofmann SG. Why cognitive behavioral therapy is the current gold standard of psychotherapy. Front Psych. 2018;9:4. https://doi.org/10.3389/fpsyt.2018.00004.
16. Ellis A. Rational psychotherapy & individual psychology. J Individ Psychol. 1957;13:38–44.
17. Engel GL. The need for a new medical model: a challenge for biomedicine. Science. 1977;196(4286):129–36.
18. Feldman JM, Matte L, Interian A, Lehrer PM, Lu SE, Scheckner B, Steinberg DM, Oken T, Kotay A, Sinha S, Shim C. Psychological treatment of comorbid asthma & panic disorder in Latino adults: results from a randomized controlled trial. Behav Res Ther. 2016;87:142–54. https://doi.org/10.1016/j.brat.2016.09.007.
19. Foa, E. B., Hembree, E. A., & Rothbaum, B. O. (2019). Prolonged exposure therapy for PTSD: emotional processing of traumatic experiences—therapist guide (2nd ed.). Oxford University Press.
20. Fraser K, Ma IWY, Teteris E, Baxter H, Wright B, McLaughlin K. Emotionally resonant moments in simulation-based education: a qualitative study. Fam Med. 2015;47(7):517–22. https://www.stfm.org/familymedicine/vol47issue7/Fraser517.
21. Gaudiano BA. Cognitive-behavioral therapies: achievements & challenges. EBMH. 2017;11(1):5–7.
22. Grenier J, Chomienne MH, Gaboury I, Ritchie P, Hogg W. Collaboration between family physicians & psychologists: what do family physicians know about psychologists' work? Can Fam Physician. 2008;54(2):232–3.
23. Hasler G, Gergen PJ, Kleinbaum DG, Ajdacic V, Gamma A, Eich D, Rössler W, Angst J. Asthma & panic in young adults: a 20-year prospective community study. Am J Respir Crit Care Med. 2005;171(11):1224–30. https://doi.org/10.1164/rccm.200412-1669OC.
24. Hayes SC, Hofmann SG. The third wave of cognitive behavioral therapy & the rise of process-based care. World Psychiatry. 2017;16(3):245–6. https://doi.org/10.1002/wps.20442.
25. Hayes SC, Strosahl KD, Wilson KG. Acceptance & commitment therapy: an experiential approach to behavior change. Guilford Press; 1999.
26. Holdgaard A, Eckhardt-Hansen C, Lassen CF, Kjesbu IE, Dall CH, Michaelsen KL, Sibilitz KL, Prescott E, Rasmusen HK. Cognitive-behavioural therapy reduces psychological distress in younger patients with cardiac disease: a randomized trial. Eur Heart J. 2023;44(11):986–96. https://doi.org/10.1093/eurheartj/ehac792.
27. Institute of Medicine (US) Committee on Sleep Medicine & Research. In: Colten HR, Altevogt BM, editors. Sleep disorders & sleep deprivation: an unmet public health problem. National Academies Press; 2006. https://www.ncbi.nlm.nih.gov/books/NBK19961/.
28. Kew KM, Nashed M, Dulay V, Yorke J. Cognitive behavioural therapy (CBT) for adults & adolescents with asthma. Cochrane Database Syst Rev. 2016;9(9):CD011818. https://doi.org/10.1002/14651858.CD011818.pub2.
29. Li Y, Buys N, Li Z, Li L, Song Q, Sun J. The efficacy of cognitive behavioral therapy-based interventions on patients with hypertension: a systematic review & meta-analysis. Prev Med Rep. 2021;23:101477. https://doi.org/10.1016/j.pmedr.2021.101477.
30. Li Y, Storch EA, Ferguson S, Li L, Buys N, Sun J. The efficacy of cognitive behavioral therapy-based intervention on patients with diabetes: a meta-analysis. Diabetes Res Clin Pract. 2022;189:109965. https://doi.org/10.1016/j.diabres.2022.109965.
31. Linehan MM. Cognitive-behavioral treatment of borderline personality disorder. Guilford Press; 1993.
32. McDaniel SH, Campbell TL, Hepworth J, Lorenz A. Family-oriented primary care. Springer Science & Business Media; 2005.
33. Mills S, Torrance N, Smith BH. Identification & management of chronic pain in primary care: a review. Curr Psychiatry Rep. 2016;18(2):22. https://doi.org/10.1007/s11920-015-0659-9.
34. Momen NC, Plana-Ripoll O, Agerbo E, Benros ME, Børglum AD, Christensen MK, Dalsgaard S, Degenhardt L, de Jonge P, Debost JPG, Fenger-Grøn M, Gunn JM, Iburg KM, Kessing

LV, Kessler RC, Laursen TM, Lim CCW, Mors O, Mortensen PB, Musliner KL, et al. Association between mental disorders & subsequent medical conditions. N Engl J Med. 2020;382(18):1721–31. https://doi.org/10.1056/NEJMoa1915784.
35. Monson CM, Shnaider P. Treating PTSD with cognitive–behavioral therapies: interventions that work. American Psychological Association; 2014.
36. National Institute of Mental Health. Mental illness. National Institutes of Health. n.d. https://www.nimh.nih.gov/health/statistics/mental-illness.
37. Pilipenko N, Chang MN. Re-imagining clinical interviewing: bridging the gap between theory & practice for equitable care. In: Bonilla-Silva E, Haozous E, Kayingo G, McDade W, Meeks L, Núñez A, Oyeyemi T, Southerland J, Sukhera J, editors. Reimagining medical education for the future of health equity & social justice. Elsevier; 2024. p. 140–54.
38. Pompoli A, Furukawa TA, Efthimiou O, Imai H, Tajika A, Salanti G. Dismantling cognitive-behaviour therapy for panic disorder: a systematic review & component network meta-analysis. Psychol Med. 2018;48(12):1945–53. https://doi.org/10.1017/S0033291717003919.
39. Resick PA, Monson CM, Chard KM. Cognitive processing therapy for PTSD: a comprehensive therapist manual. 2nd ed. The Guilford Press; 2017.
40. Rikard SM, Strahan AE, Schmit KM, Guy GP Jr. Chronic pain among adults—United States, 2019–2021. MMWR Morb Mortal Wkly Rep. 2023;72(15):379–85. https://doi.org/10.15585/mmwr.mm7215a1.
41. Rousseau DM, Gunia BC. Evidence-based practice: the psychology of EBP implementation. Annu Rev Psychol. 2016;67:667–92. https://doi.org/10.1146/annurev-psych-122414-03333.
42. Sackett DL, Rosenberg WM, Gray JA, Haynes RB, Richardson WS. Evidence based medicine: what it is & what it isn't. BMJ. 1996;312(7023):71–2. https://doi.org/10.1136/bmj.312.7023.71.
43. Segal ZV, Williams JMG, Teasdale JD. Mindfulness-based cognitive therapy for depression: a new approach to preventing relapse. Guilford Press; 2002.
44. Society of Clinical Psychology, Division 12, American Psychological Association. Treatments. n.d. https://div12.org/treatments/?_sfm_related_diagnosis=8149.
45. Tobin. Psychology.org. Psychology licensing requirements in New York. 2025. https://www.psychology.org/psychology/licensure/new-york/.
46. Upshur CC, Luckmann RS, Savageau JA. Primary care provider concerns about management of chronic pain in community clinic populations. J Gen Intern Med. 2006;21(6):652–5. https://doi.org/10.1111/j.1525-1497.2006.00412.x.
47. van Straten A, van der Zweerde T, Kleiboer A, Cuijpers P, Morin CM, Lancee J. Cognitive & behavioral therapies in the treatment of insomnia: a meta-analysis. Sleep Med Rev. 2018;38:3–16. https://doi.org/10.1016/j.smrv.2017.02.001.

Index

N. Pilipenko, K. M. Desai (eds.), *8 Conditions Primary Care Clinicians Dread to Treat*, https://doi.org/10.1007/978-3-032-12819-5

V

W

Y

GPSR Compliance

The European Union's (EU) General Product Safety Regulation (GPSR) is a set of rules that requires consumer products to be safe and our obligations to ensure this.

If you have any concerns about our products, you can contact us on ProductSafety@springernature.com

In case Publisher is established outside the EU, the EU authorized representative is:

Springer Nature Customer Service Center GmbH
Europaplatz 3
69115 Heidelberg, Germany

Batch number: 10370708

Printed by Printforce, the Netherlands